HABITS, NOT DIETS
The Real Way to Weight Control

James M. Ferguson
M.D.

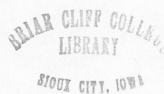

BULL PUBLISHING COMPANY

P.O. Box 208
Palo Alto, California 94302

Copyright 1976
Bull Publishing Co.

ISBN 0-915950-06-5

Library of Congress Catalog No. 76-4098

Cover design: Jill Casty
Back cover photo: George Chang

Contents

Maintenance Weeks 1–5

PREFACE

The last ten years have witnessed a marked change in our views about the eating which leads to obesity. The origins of such eating had long been assumed to lie in some defective inner state, metabolic or psychological, and the control of obesity lay in the remedying of that defect. The result was a vast outpouring of appetite-suppressant medication and a no less intense program of exhorting obese people to exercise will power and self-denial.

Two developments shifted our attention from defects within the person to the social environment around him. One was understanding the powerful influence of social factors on obesity. The other was the introduction of behavior modification.

The application of behavior modification to the treatment of obesity was a natural. For it is ideally suited to analyzing just how social factors exert their influence, and it has proceeded to do just that. Only eight years after its introduction, a short time in the history of psychotherapy research, behavior modification has sparked a veritable explosion of research on the treatment of obesity. Within the past four years alone, over 30 reports have been devoted to applications of behavior modification in this area. They have established beyond a doubt these techniques are more effective than traditional weight reduction measures; and they are elucidating just which of the many behavioral techniques are the most effective.

The explosion of research on behavior modification of obesity has been paralleled by an enormous increase of interest on the part of the lay public. Research results have found their way with increasing frequency into the popular press, and treatment programs based upon behavioral principles are consistently over-subscribed. The demand for help in the control of obesity has even led to the recent publication of self-help manuals based upon behavioral principles and presented in the form of programmed texts.

In this climate of high expectations and limited treatment resources, the program developed by Dr. Ferguson may be particularly useful. It is based upon a sound background of research, tempered by intensive clinical testing designed to refine and polish the most effective techniques and to ascertain the optimal order of their presentation. During the past several months I have had occasion to use Dr. Ferguson's program and have found it very well-suited to the treatment of the majority of obese people who have come to the Stanford Eating Disorders Clinic.

The program is particularly effective in its presentation of techniques which fall into the general category of stimulus control. Many of these techniques are a matter of common sense and have been in common use in weight reduction efforts in the past: for example, developing the automatic habit of making low-calorie foods like celery and raw carrots readily available. Persons who have used such techniques in the past are thereby encouraged to try them again while newcomers are exposed to these time-tested maneuvers. Other techniques may be new to overweight persons. A particularly effective one, developed from theories on stimulus control, is the establishment of a "designated eating place," where all food, meals and snacks alike, are to be consumed.

A key feature of any behavior modification program, and one which is particularly well exemplified in Dr. Ferguson's program, is the use of feedback about performance. A cornerstone of behavioral programs has been the use of a Food Diary to help people become aware of what they eat and the circumstances under which they eat. They are invaluable in helping people to define problem times, places and circumstances of over-eating. They may even by themselves reduce eating; at times it is simpler not to eat than to have to write down what one has eaten.

This program contains a number of innovative forms of feedback beyond the Food Diary. The "Eating Place Record" provides useful information about the extent to which the person is achieving the goal of confining all eating to the "designated eating place." The "Behavioral Analysis Form" depicts progress made in cutting down on snacking and confining eating to mealtimes. The use of "an eating ratio" provides feedback on the rate of eating, valuable information in helping to reduce its speed.

A deceptively simple form of feedback is built into one of the most effective behavioral control measures in the program. This is pre-planning of meals and snacks. Writing down exactly what will be eaten during one or more meals on the following day provides strong incentives to eat these foods and to resist impulse eating. Pre-planned foods are written in one color of ink, the actual foods consumed in another. The decreasing amount of two-colored Diary pages is a reassuring reminder of progress to date and problems to be overcome.

Many of the techniques utilized in this and other behavioral programs for obesity are standard ones based upon problems which are found among most overweight people. Each person, however, has problems which are specific to him, and Dr. Ferguson's program provides guidance in identifying such problems and in coping with them. Such problem-solving exercises are among the most attractive features of this program.

Another special virtue of this program lies in the five-week "Maintenance" periods which follow five-week periods of active instruction. The large number of new techniques introduced in most behavioral programs often overload the participant and result in less than optimal exercise of the behaviors which are learned. The Maintenance periods devoted to practice of the still-imperfectly learned techniques provide a splendid opportunity for the firm establishment of these behaviors, before being subjected to the pressures of extensive new learning.

Behavior modification is no panacea. It demands of participants a great deal of hard work and often major changes in personal habits and life situations. But for those who succeed, the results are well worth the effort. For behavioral programs can lead not only to the control of obesity, but also to a more rewarding inner-directed life.

Albert J. Stunkard, M.D.

ACKNOWLEDGEMENTS

The work of many scientists has contributed to the preparation of this manual. Techniques have been incorporated from a wide variety of sources—psychology, psychiatry, medicine, physiology, and common sense. Although many of the individual investigators in the field of appetite and weight control are mentioned in the bibliography, there are countless others who have made significant contributions to the body of information from which this text has been developed. Without this basic research carried out by hundreds of individuals working in many scientific disciplines, there would be no effective control of obesity.

I would like to specifically express my gratitude to two great teachers and friends, Dr. Albert J. Stunkard and Dr. W. Stewart Agras. Without their help, encouragement, and continued interest, this book would probably not have been started and certainly would have never been finished.

The clinical program from which this text evolved was repeatedly tested and revised at the Stanford Eating Disorders Clinic in the Department of Psychiatry and Behavioral Sciences at Stanford Medical School. Evaluation groups were conducted and the program critiqued by a number of friends, many of whom are now widely dispersed from Stanford. These include: Billie Bem, M.S.W., Children's Hospital, San Francisco; Stan Chapman, Ph.D., Emory University; Carlos C. Greaves, M.D., Centro Médico Docente La Trinidad, Caracas, Venezuela; Brandon Qualls, M.D., Brown University; Colleen Rand, Ph.D., Stanford University; Jan Ruby, Stanford University; C.B. Taylor, M.D., University of Utah Medical School; Roger Walsh, M.D., Ph.D., Stanford University; Joellen Werene, M.D., Stanford University, and Carolyn Wright, B.A., University of California San Diego Medical School. I want to express my appreciation to each of them for their critical feedback and many words of encouragement when they were sorely needed.

The patients who used the program at Stanford contributed immeasurably to its development. Their participation ranged from the reinforcement I felt when they lost weight to their many helpful suggestions about format and style. A final thanks goes to Dave Bull, who has patiently guided me through the maze of publication, and to my wife and children who have waited for me at home on those many evenings when I have been at the clinic teaching people to change their eating habits.

Introduction

This manual is for your use in your individual weight control program. It is written to be read in weekly installments. You are encouraged to take notes in the manual, and to underline points which are significant to you or which have special meaning in your life situation. Use it as a workbook.

The manual was initially written for use by the Stanford University Eating Disorders Clinic. It is based on theories developed in many different areas of psychology, and if used as written, it can be very effective in helping you control your eating behaviors—and consequently your weight.

Most people find that the written material continues to be useful long after the twenty weeks are over. If three months, a year, or five years from now you find your eating is getting out of control, take out your manual, fill out a food diary for a few weeks, and choose the appropriate techniques to correct whatever problems are leading to your over-eating. These exercises will be as valid five years from now as they are today.

If you do not understand any of the materials presented in the lessons, re-read them until they make sense. Self-examination sections are included throughout the text to make you stop and think, and to help point out ideas that might be conceptually difficult. If you find you are answering some of the questions ''no,'' re-read the lesson. It is essential that you have a good understanding of the theory and homework presented at each lesson as you progress through the program.

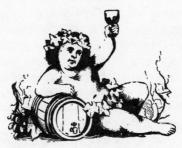

Lesson One

Introduction to the Behavioral Control of Weight—Habit Awareness

WEIGH-IN.

Weigh yourself and record your weight on the Master Data Sheet located at the end of this text. Since this is the first piece of information on the Data Sheet, it is important that you put it in the correct place on the form. Today there will be no weight change to calculate. The large dot at the top of the diagonal line on the graph paper indicates the starting point for your weight graph.

INTRODUCTION TO THE PROGRAM.

You are beginning this behavioral program to learn how to control your weight. During the next twenty weeks you will work to change your eating habits. Your weight, which brought you to this program, will be one of the ways you measure how effective you are at changing your eating habits. The more they change and the more you are able to control your eating behaviors, the more weight you will lose.

Today you have begun by weighing yourself and recording your weight on the Master Data Sheet. Each week you will repeat this process, as close to the same time of day as possible. Next week you will add the additional step of calculating and graphing your weight change on the Master Data Sheet. (In subsequent weeks you will calculate first the weight change during the week, then the cumulative weight change since the beginning of the program.) This will help you see exactly how well your weight change program is progressing each week. The diagonal line across the graph on your Master Data Sheet shows a weight loss of one pound a week. You may lose faster or more slowly, or your rate of loss may change from week to week. Everyone loses at a different rate! The diagonal line will keep reminding you of how your rate of weight loss compares with the one-pound-per-week rate which we have arbitrarily chosen for you to compare yourself to. Figure 1 shows how a complete weight graph looks. It reflects the cumulative weekly weight loss of individuals in an actual behavioral weight control group.

Each lesson begins with a weighing, and then homework correction. The homework is designed to be completed in one-week blocks. To use the program most effectively, *you should not go faster* than one lesson each week.

A reward system has been built into the program to help you stay motivated to finish all ten lessons and do all of the homework. Set aside twenty-five dollars today for a personal reward. It should be separated from other funds, and kept segregated from the money you deal with regularly; ideally, it should be removed from your control. Lock it away, or give it to someone else to hold for you. This is your reward money. (The $25.00 is not a magic figure; it should be an amount that you can afford, but which is meaningful for you. There is no rule that you or someone else can't "up the ante," if you feel you want to work for higher stakes.)

At the end of the book you will find a Homework Credit Sheet which shows the refund value of each piece of homework. For each lesson you will be asked to complete all of the homework, even when you may feel that you don't need it or that it is busy work. For credit, all that counts is that you have done the homework. There are no right or wrong answers. Give yourself full credit towards a refund if you complete the homework forms each week. At the end of 15 weeks you will total up the amount of credit you have earned, and you will pay yourself that amount of money. It should be yours to spend as you see fit, preferably

FIGURE 1. WEEKLY WEIGHT LOSS FOR INDIVIDUAL MEMBERS OF A BEHAVIORAL WEIGHT CONTROL GROUP

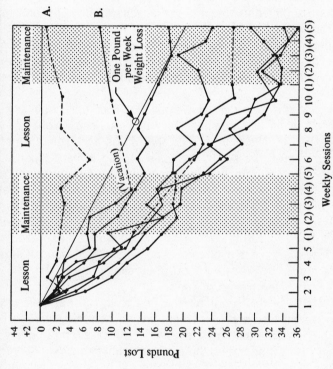

Each group member is represented by one line. Broken lines indicate missed meetings, and shaded areas represent Maintenance weeks. Patient A was a businessman who could not attend meetings regularly; Patient B went on vacation during the second half of the course.

on yourself. Any extra unearned deposit should be given away—to a worthy cause, or even more motivating, to a cause you do not believe in (for example, a liberal Democrat making a donation to the John Birch Society).

INTRODUCTION TO THE BEHAVIORAL
CONTROL OF WEIGHT—HABIT AWARENESS.

Throughout history many methods have been tried for losing weight. Between them the popular press and the medical profession have probably suggested several hundred. These have been based mainly on drugs and diets, although such techniques as hypnosis, psychotherapy, and surgery have also had their advocates. Most of these methods work spectacularly for a few people, but not very well for most. Of those people who do lose weight, most regain it. I'm sure you have had this frustrating experience; that is one of the reasons you have decided to try "behavior modification."

This program is aimed at weight loss, but only indirectly. With behavior modification you are specifically trying to lose weight *as a result* of behavior change. The main reason that drugs and diets are not very effective in the long run is that their use is time limited. When a drug or diet is over, most people resume their old patterns of eating and regain their weight. This is especially true for individuals in stressful situations, or people with chaotic life styles. Regaining weight does not mean that they are weak-willed, or not trying. But while they were losing weight they did not learn to eat in a more sensible manner; their eating habits (or eating behavior) did not change, and when they found themselves back in the real world with real food, they simply ate in the same way they had always eaten before.

The object of this program is to teach you to eat in a way that will lead to weight loss and permanent weight control. Although it may take more of your time than a series of shots or pills, and in many ways is more demanding than a diet, there are real advantages to this method. A follow-up survey of patients in the University of Pennsylvania program showed that of those who lost 20 or more pounds (over 50 percent of the original group), more than 80 percent were able to keep that weight off for over two years.[1]

It is impossible to make any reliable promises as to the outcome of this program. It will depend entirely on you. Some people do extremely well; others never become fully engaged in the program, or are unwilling or unable to put the time and effort into the individual lessons, and as a consequence, they do not lose as much weight. (Weight loss is important for your morale, and it is an indicator of how much progress you are making; but once again, it's worthwhile emphasizing that the primary goal is behavior change.) Used with groups, this program has resulted in an average loss of about 1 pound per week for each group member. Some people are able to lose twice this fast.

Control of eating habits (and consequent weight loss) is largely a matter of establishing priorities. If it is not important for you to lose weight, you won't. To follow this program and to be successful takes time and effort. You will be expected to take more time eating than you do now, to experience food more thoroughly, and to enjoy everything you eat. If you cannot spare the time to really eat, your program will probably be unsuccessful.

There are many theories explaining why people become obese, some of which apply to only a few individuals. For most people who are overweight, the cause is unknown. In 99 percent of the cases, exhaustive medical tests and investigation will be negative; no specific cause can be found for the weight problems. Only in few cases can the cause of obesity be identified. These have included thyroid, pituitary, or adrenal malfunction, varieties of diabetes, tumors (rare), and very uncommon neurological disorders. There are also the general factors of the tendency of everyone to put on weight as he or she grows older (caloric need decreases with age), and inherited tendencies to be overweight. The latter factor is difficult to separate from environmental learning because eating habits tend to be very similar among members of the same family.

Many therapists still adhere to personality trait theories and believe that overweight individuals have deep-seated psychological problems, which are compensated for by eating, or emotional states which are represented by an "equivalent in eating behaviors." Research has shown that individuals with "deep-seated psychological problems" rarely lose weight with traditional treatments like psychoanalysis, despite greater insight into their problems. The problems are probably not the cause of the obesity.

Finally, there is the theory that individuals who became obese when they were young acquired too many fat cells as a result of over-eating in early childhood. There is good evidence for this theory, and it can be a permanent handicap for anyone fighting weight problems, but it does not make weight loss impossible. The ultimate cause of obesity is more energy taken into your body than is used. If this imbalance can be corrected, if you become able to take in fewer calories than you burn up each day, your overweight problem will be corrected, regardless of its cause.

(At this point, and regularly throughout this book, you will be asked to pause and reflect—and to re-read parts you find are unclear.)

Is everything clear?

- Do you see why it is necessary to learn new behaviors to keep weight off? Yes_____ No_____
- What goes wrong with diets, pills, and other weight control methods?

  1. _____

  2. _____

Over-eating and inactivity are behavior patterns that have been learned and practiced for years. Like all firmly entrenched habits, they continue because they pay off. Relief of hunger is one of the most obvious rewards for eating; but I think that after reflecting a bit you will be able to think of many situations in which you eat which are not related to hunger.

For example, many people eat in response to anger, happiness, sadness, fatigue, insomnia, social pressure, and boredom. Because there are so many influences on your eating habits, because you have *learned* to eat in response to so many situations, these eating behaviors are very hard to change. It takes a thorough and systematic program of working on almost every aspect of your life to free you from all of the stimuli that tell you to eat.

Thinking of eating behaviors as learned is quite an optimistic way to look at the problem of being overweight. If you have excess pounds because of a learned habit, then the solution seems obvious—you have to learn a new set of behaviors to take the place of the old ones. You have to eat in a new way. It may be necessary to pursue this retraining to the point of actually learning a new way of putting your food in your mouth! As you establish new eating habits, you will notice that almost automatically the old patterns which are no longer practiced gradually fade away.

It is very important to understand that the goals of this program are *not* to stop eating, or simply to diet, but to develop a new set of eating habits, so that when you lose weight, it stays off. This involves not only what foods you eat, but also how, when, where, and with whom you eat, and the circumstances under which you acquire food.

This program does not focus on increasing will power and trying to resist food, but on rearranging the environment, and in this way producing changes in your own behavior. For example, if you always respond to the sight of pretzels by first going on a binge of eating the pretzels and then progressing to other snacks, it doesn't make any sense to fight with "will power." The more direct way is to remove the pretzels. If you never see pretzels, you will lose the habit.

Research has shown that overweight people are more sensitive to many aspects of their environment than their thin counterparts.[2] This increased sensitivity is a mixed blessing. People who are overweight are more likely to respond to external cues, such as the sight or smell of food, a television ad, the time of day, or a certain place at home which has been associated with food—by eating. At the same time they are less likely to respond to internal cues for eating, like hunger. Working to change the external world pays off—it removes many of these cues, and teaches you ways of dealing with some of them you cannot change, like time of day, or social situations.

Do You See How This Applies to You?

• Have you ever thought you might be more sensitive to stimuli or cues to eat than the people around you? Yes _____
No_____

• Do you eat when you are not hungry? Yes_____ No_____

• What are some of the things or cues that start you eating?

1. _____

2. _____

3. _____

• Do you see how learning a new set of behaviors and rearranging the world around you a little bit can help you avoid some of those cues or reminders to eat? Yes_____ No_____

In this program the focus will be on strengthening "good" eating habits rather than trying to weaken "bad" ones. The reason for this is simple: It is easier to learn a new habit than to try to forget an old one. Furthermore, if you can make the new habit incompatible with the old one, the old habit will naturally decrease in strength, since the two cannot happen at the same time. For example, it is impossible to wolf down a meal in a few minutes if you put your fork down after each bite.

One of the first things you will do in this program is to develop *habit awareness.* You will examine in detail your present eating habits and determine the specific behaviors that are leading to your present weight problem. Once you have identified these behaviors, you will proceed to figure out which environmental conditions control them. Finally, you will be in a position to make changes in your environment which will encourage the new behaviors that you are striving for.

Changing any habit—smoking, drinking, eating—is very hard, especially if you try to do it all at once. The way around the difficulty is to break the behavior you want to change into parts, e.g., shopping, preparing food, identification of where and when you eat, etc., and to work on each part, one at a time. This makes the going slow, but when you begin to feel that things are too slow, remember how many years it took your present way of eating to evolve, and how much faster (albeit over several months) this program will be. You are trying to reverse and substitute for some of the strongest behaviors in your daily life. To try to change them overnight would only invite failure. The way to succeed is to take small steps and to practice each one until it is "over learned," until it seems second nature, until it is a habit.

Some weeks you will be presented techniques for altering your eating environment which you will be able to learn and master readily. Other weeks the lesson may introduce a behavioral control technique that is difficult for you. This is inevitable. If necessary, take a couple of weeks extra to master any step that seems especially difficult for you—don't try to go too fast or jump ahead. You will only be courting failure.

Changing behaviors takes time, and your weight loss in this twenty-week program may not be what you hoped for at the beginning. I can sympathize with this and wish there were a magic way to produce changes —there isn't. It takes time and a lot of effort to change, and at this point the last thing you need is moralizing about being overweight—to put the book down, to feel guilty, and perhaps to say, "to hell with it."

You may not be able to master some of the techniques. That's O.K. There is no race and no competition. The object is not to make you feel bad, but to help you control the stimuli that cause you to over-eat. Although nothing would be lost by going on a sensible diet while you are involved in this program (you would learn just as much about behavior control and you would probably lose weight faster), the choice of whether to include a diet is yours. This program does *not* include a diet; the purpose is to learn to eat *anything,* but with control.

Weight loss is *not* a behavior. You have begun this program to change your eating behaviors, and you should not judge your progress solely by weight loss. As you know, weight loss can occur for a variety of reasons. In most weight loss programs, with weight loss as the sole criterion for success, people are subtly encouraged to do anything to lose weight before they weigh in. They starve themselves for the day, or use laxatives or diuretics before they are weighed. You should strive for weight loss as a result of changed eating habits. Each week you will check your weight and at the same time you will be grading your homework as a way of checking your progress with your eating behaviors. Ultimately you will be your own weight control expert, and you will monitor your eating habits automatically. Weight will become a secondary concern. The value of the educational approach we will be using is that once you have learned the principles and techniques of self-management, you will be able to apply them to all of the situations to which you are exposed. There will be no more going on and off of diets.

By learning new eating habits and losing weight you will find that people react to you differently, that your self-image will change, and that you will enjoy eating more. Every pattern of behavior has its consequences. Over-eating leads to a change in body size, a poor self-image, a loss of mobility, etc. This, in turn, leads to a loss of self-esteem, and often depression. Changing eating patterns can affect many aspects of your life, and you can expect to have different experiences in the world. These experiences, e.g., being accepted by others, being admired, etc., can in turn lead to changes in your way of thinking and your feelings about yourself.

As you lose weight, expect changes to take place in other areas of your life. If you are threatened by looking thin, by looking sexier, by looking more athletic, or by receiving compliments about such things, think twice about losing weight. If you are not bothered by these thoughts, enjoy them. The rewards for weight loss are not immediate. It takes time for the health, appearance, and social benefits. On the other hand, eating has an immediate reward which sometimes makes it difficult to remember the long-term benefits of not eating until it is too late. By taking small steps, adding small behavior changes each week, it is possible to change. Eating skills, like any other skills, take time to develop and perfect.

You have total responsibility for yourself in this program. Although you want to lose weight, to do so you have to be willing to make some difficult changes in your eating habits. Some of these changes may seem silly in a social context, such as putting your fork down between bites. To solve this conflict you have to assign priorities to your behaviors and try to avoid the trap of saying, ''That's a good idea, but I could never do it because. . . .'' When this happens, you have to ask yourself, ''What are my priorities? . . .'' For example, is not being able to spend time eating breakfast more important than losing weight? There are no right and wrong answers, and at some point behavior change and weight reduction may not be as high on your list of priorities as other behaviors, such as getting to work early, or taking only five minutes for lunch between assignments.

Weight reduction is not easy, but it doesn't have to be painful, or even a hungry experience. It is a long-term project, and it will be successful only on that basis. Short term gains and losses are relatively unimportant. To make this program work, it is important that you understand the principles, both now at the start, and when new ideas are introduced. Even when you understand each technique and are satisfied that you can apply that technique to your life, your work is not finished. It is essential that you *practice,* until these techniques become habits.

Part of every behavior program is the concept of measurement. You need to know where you stand in terms of current behaviors, to know whether or not the behavior changes you have introduced have been effective. The period of observation before any changes are introduced is called "the baseline." During this period you collect information about a particular habit or set of behaviors that you want to change or modify. When you have become aware of your eating habits, during a week of baseline observation, you will be able to see eating patterns that can be easily changed. The following week's observation will tell you if you have been successful in modifying the behaviors you identified during the baseline period.

In this program a great deal of emphasis is placed on keeping records of eating behaviors, both to tell you what you are doing now, and to enable you to see when a change has occurred. The first measure you will be keeping is a Daily Food Diary. The purpose of this record is habit awareness: to make you aware of how you eat and to gather baseline information about your eating habits.

One of the first things you will notice during the coming week is that accurately keeping the Diary will make you acutely aware of everything you eat. The natural tendency will be to decrease the amount of your intake, to question yourself each time you begin to eat, and to question each food portion you are considering eating. One of the benefits of this increased awareness will be a delay between impulse and action—you will stop and think. Initially this may be more in the form of, "I don't want to write this down, it's too much work and easier just not to eat it." Eventually this type of internal dialogue will change to something more like, "I really don't want to eat that; I'm not hungry now."

The Food Diary has several columns which ask you to report on different behaviors and feelings. The column headings will change from week to week as the emphasis of the lessons changes; however, a Food Diary in some form will be part of each lesson.

Let's Review a Bit

- Do you understand the theory of behavior change? Yes_____ No_____ (If you answered No, re-read this chapter.)

- Do you see why this is a slow program? Yes_____ No_____

- Why does it have to be slow—why take small steps? (To insure success.)

- Why are self-observation and homework so important?

_____

(Homework and self-observation are the only ways you have of assessing behavior change; you cannot measure eating behaviors directly. Even your weight each week is only an indirect measure of changed behavior.)

- Do you understand why behavior change and weight loss have to be high priority items in your life if this program is going to work?

_____

(Because you will be tempted to give up, or to pick and choose techniques.)

HOMEWORK

Among the materials for today's lesson you will find a sample of a filled-in Food Diary and seven blank Food Diary forms. They are divided horizontally by lines that represent 6:00 a.m., 11:00 a.m., 4:00 p.m., and 9:00 p.m. These lines separate your eating into four time categories. In the first vertical column you record the actual starting time for each meal or snack. In the next column, mark down the length in minutes of each meal or snack. Mark an "M" or "S" in the third column, depending on whether it is a meal or snack, and rate that eating episode on a scale of 0 to 3 in the "H" column to indicate the degree of your hunger: "0" indicates no hunger, or the feeling you have after a large meal; "1" is some hunger; "2" is normal hunger; "3" is equivalent to the hungriest you have ever been.

Describe your body position by a number code: "1"—walking, "2"—standing, "3"—sitting, "4"—lying down. In the Activity column, indicate activities carried out while eating; for example, watching television, reading the paper, or working. "Location of eating" asks for a short description of where you eat the meal or snack; for example, "car," "desk," "kitchen table."

In the next column, indicate the content of your meal or snack, by kind of food and quantity. The purpose of the quantity description is to give yourself feedback on the amount of food you eat. Choose units of measurement that you will be able to duplicate from week to week. It doesn't matter whether you describe food portions by ounces, servings, cups, or handfuls, as long as it always indicates roughly the same amount of food. The remaining columns are designed to collect information about two food-related behaviors.

Save your completed Food Diaries. The information on them will be used in future lessons.

The second form for this week's homework is a sheet of graph paper. Draw a rough plan of your house on this piece of paper. Precision is not as important as completeness in including such food-related objects as your television set, desk, telephone, table, refrigerator, etc. During the next week, put a small "M" or "S" at the appropriate places on the plan to mark where you eat each meal or snack. This will give you a picture of how random or spread out your eating places are at home. If you want to involve the family, or feel that their eating or snacking behaviors influence you, you can suggest that they mark the same graph with a different color. In this way, you can make a map for the whole family's eating pattern for a week. (Again, as will be the case each time a new form is introduced, there is a filled-in sample form before the blank form which you are to use.)

Each week you will have homework similar to today's. You will check your homework next week and record whether or not it was completed on your Homework Credit schedule. Each week you will credit a portion of your $25 homework deposit to yourself for each part of the homework assignment completed. This small amount of money often makes the difference between carrying out assignments and forgetting to do them. It is a good feeling to finish the program 20 pounds lighter and 25 dollars richer.

A final suggestion to help increase the probability of success: Involve someone else in your behavior change program. Teach your lessons to your spouse, children, neighbors, co-workers, schoolmates, or anyone you see regularly. This will not only help them understand what you are going through, but it will also give you a chance to consolidate your learning when you put all of the instructional materials into your own words to teach someone else. Most people are eager to be included. Soon you may find you have started a class of your own. Teaching others can only benefit your own personal weight control program.

In summary, most eating patterns are learned behaviors. The way to control weight and maintain weight loss is not through dieting. This program is not a diet, it is a method to control your environment and the stimuli that cause you to eat in a way that results in weight loss. By systematically applying a wide variety of behavior therapy techniques, it is possible to learn new patterns of eating behaviors. These changes must be introduced a small step at a time.

In many ways changing eating habits is like playing the piano. To expect anything more than scales and exercises at first would be silly. By the end of this course, we hope to have you playing Mozart.

Consider What You Have Read.

- If you have a question about any aspect of the homework, the Food Diary, or the House Plan, re-read the relevant part of the text. It is very important that you understand each step as you go along.

INSTRUCTIONS FOR FILLING OUT THE FOOD DIARY — Week One

Time: starting time for a meal or snack.

Minutes spent eating: length of the eating episode in minutes.

M/S: meal or snack: indicate type of eating by the appropriate letter, "M" or "S".

H: hunger on a scale of 0 to 3.   0 = no hunger, 3 = extreme hunger

Body position: 1 — walking
                     2 — standing
                     3 — sitting
                     4 — lying down

Activity while eating: Record any activity you carry out while eating, such as
    watching television, reading, or sweeping the floor.

Location of eating: Record each place you eat; for example your car, kitchen table,
    or living room couch.

Food type and quantity: Indicate the content of your meal or snack by kind of food
    and quantity. Choose units of measurement that you will be able to reproduce
    from week to week. Accuracy is not as important as consistency.

Eating with whom: Indicate with whom you are eating, or if you are eating that
    meal or snack alone.

Feelings before and during eating: Record your feelings or mood immediately before
    or during eating. Typical feelings are angry, bored, confused, depressed,
    frustrated, sad, etc. Many times you will have no feelings associated with eating.
    In this case, write down "none".

FOOD DIARY – Lesson One

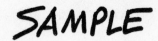

Day of Week __MONDAY__   Name__C. B. T.__

Time	Minutes Spent Eating	M/S	H	Body Position	Activity While Eating	Location Of Eating	Food Type and Quantity	Eating With Whom	Feeling While Eating
6:00									
7:20-7:30	10 MIN	M	O	3	PAPER	KITCHEN	COFFEE CEREAL	WIFE	NONE
8:15-8:20	5 MIN	S	O	2	TALKING	WORK	DONUT COFFEE	FRIENDS	TIRED
10:30-?	5 MIN	S	1	1	WALKING	HALL	DONUT	ALONE	LATE
11:00									
12:30	1 MIN	S	2	2	WORK	DESK	CANDY BAR	ALONE	LATE
3:30-3:40	10 MIN	M	3	3	READING	RESTAUR.	HAMBURG.	ALONE	TIRED
4:00									
5:30-6:00	½ HR	S	3	3	PAPER TV	L.R.	SCOTCH/ WATER NUTS	FAMILY	TIRED
6:00-7:00	1 HR	M	2	3	TV	DR.	BEEF TV DINNER ICE CREAM	FAMILY	ANGRY
9:00									
10:30-10:45	15 MIN	S	O	2	TV	LR	ICE CREAM	WIFE	BORED

M/S: Meal or Snack H: Degree of Hunger (0 = None, 3 = Maximum)
Body Position: 1 = Walking, 2 = Standing, 3 = Sitting, 4 = Lying Down

FOOD DIARY – Lesson One

Day of Week _____   Name_____

Time	Minutes Spent Eating	M/S	H	Body Position	Activity While Eating	Location Of Eating	Food Type and Quantity	Eating With Whom	Feeling While Eating
6:00									
11:00									
4:00									
9:00									

M/S: Meal or Snack H: Degree of Hunger (0 = None, 3 = Maximum)
Body Position: 1 = Walking, 2 = Standing, 3 = Sitting, 4 = Lying Down

FOOD DIARY -- Lesson One

Day of Week _____   Name_____

Time	Minutes Spent Eating	M/S	H	Body Position	Activity While Eating	Location Of Eating	Food Type and Quantity	Eating With Whom	Feeling While Eating
6:00									
11:00									
4:00									
9:00									

M/S: Meal or Snack H: Degree of Hunger (0 = None, 3 = Maximum)
Body Position: 1 = Walking, 2 = Standing, 3 = Sitting, 4 = Lying Down

FOOD DIARY – Lesson One

Day of Week _____   Name_____

Time	Minutes Spent Eating	M/S	H	Body Position	Activity While Eating	Location Of Eating	Food Type and Quantity	Eating With Whom	Feeling While Eating
6:00									
11:00									
4:00									
9:00									

M/S: Meal or Snack H: Degree of Hunger (0 = None, 3 = Maximum)
Body Position: 1 = Walking, 2 = Standing, 3 = Sitting, 4 = Lying Down

FOOD DIARY – Lesson One

Day of Week _____   Name _____

Time	Minutes Spent Eating	M/S	H	Body Position	Activity While Eating	Location Of Eating	Food Type and Quantity	Eating With Whom	Feeling While Eating
6:00									
11:00									
4:00									
9:00									

M/S: Meal or Snack H: Degree of Hunger (0 = None, 3 = Maximum)
Body Position: 1 = Walking, 2 = Standing, 3 = Sitting, 4 = Lying Down

FOOD DIARY – Lesson One

Day of Week _____   Name_____

Time	Minutes Spent Eating	M/S	H	Body Position	Activity While Eating	Location Of Eating	Food Type and Quantity	Eating With Whom	Feeling While Eating
6:00									
11:00									
4:00									
9:00									

M/S: Meal or Snack H: Degree of Hunger (0 = None, 3 = Maximum)
Body Position: 1 = Walking, 2 = Standing, 3 = Sitting, 4 = Lying Down

FOOD DIARY — Lesson One

Day of Week _____   Name_____

Time	Minutes Spent Eating	M/S	H	Body Position	Activity While Eating	Location Of Eating	Food Type and Quantity	Eating With Whom	Feeling While Eating
6:00									
11:00									
4:00									
9:00									

M/S: Meal or Snack H: Degree of Hunger (0 = None, 3 = Maximum)
Body Position: 1 = Walking, 2 = Standing, 3 = Sitting, 4 = Lying Down

FOOD DIARY – Lesson One

Day of Week _____   Name_____

Time	Minutes Spent Eating	M/S	H	Body Position	Activity While Eating	Location Of Eating	Food Type and Quantity	Eating With Whom	Feeling While Eating
6:00									
11:00									
4:00									
9:00									

M/S: Meal or Snack H: Degree of Hunger (0 = None, 3 = Maximum)
Body Position: 1 = Walking, 2 = Standing, 3 = Sitting, 4 = Lying Down

SAMPLE

HOUSE PLAN

PATIO
SSSS

DEN
MMMM SSSS
MMMM SSSS
M MMM
MM

FOOD X

FOOD
X

X
FOOD

KITCHEN
SS

FOOD
X

DINING ROOM
MM

LIVING ROOM

ENTRANCE HALL

MY BEDROOM

STUDY – DESK
SSS
SSS

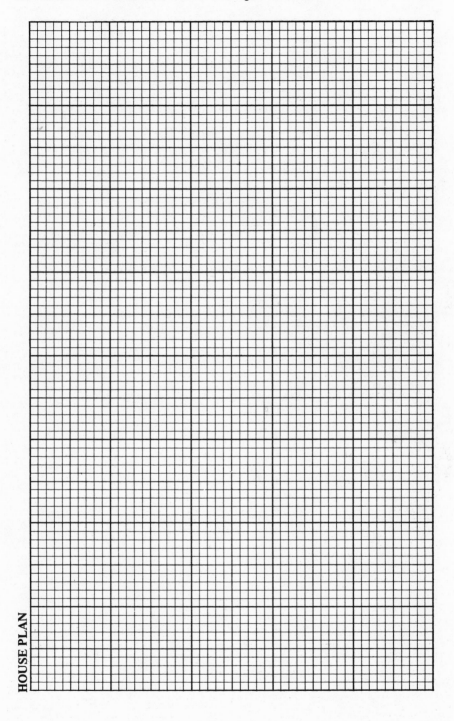

HOUSE PLAN

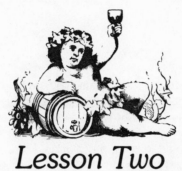

Lesson Two

Cue Elimination

WEIGH-IN AND HOMEWORK.

Weigh yourself and record your weight on your Master Data Sheet at the end of the book. Fill in your weight change since the first lesson. (Subtract today's weight from last week's weight.) Place this figure in the boxes labeled "Weight Change" and "Total Weight Change." Make a mark on the line at the top of the Master Data Sheet labeled "Week Two" to indicate the weight change for the past week. To graph your weight change, connect that mark with the dot on the line labeled "Week One."

This procedure will be repeated each week, with your weight, change of weight, and graphed difference recorded on your Master Data Sheet.

Check your homework for Lesson One and record whether or not you completed it on the Homework Credit schedule at the end of the book·

—Lesson One Food Diary complete? Yes_____ No_____
—House Plan? Yes_____ No_____

Briefly read back over your Diaries for each day and check to see if you completed them. If you had any problems filling them out, refer back to the initial instructions. In addition, see if you can identify any unusual eating patterns, things to work on during the program (like pizza six times a week), but do not make a detailed analysis of the food items or patterns of behavior. Check the House Plan to make sure it has been completed. Indicate which portions of the homework you have completed, by initialling the appropriate square on the Homework Credit schedule. This will determine the amount of money you will have earned at Lesson Ten.

REVIEW.

This is a behavior modification program. You are learning self-management techniques to change and control your eating behaviors. The ultimate goal of this course is to apply these techniques to your life in such a way that you lose weight. Weight loss *per se* is not the main objective at this point. You should lose weight, but as a result of behavior change. One of the basic points stressed in Lesson One was that this is *not* a program designed to increase "will power." If you learn new eating habits, the strength of old ones will slowly decrease. There will be no need to struggle with "will power." Your task is not to stop eating, but to eat differently.

Changing behaviors, especially those as ingrained as eating behaviors, takes time. Years of practice have formed these habits and they are often immediately rewarding. As a result, they cannot be unlearned overnight. This lesson introduces a general principle of behavior modification and shows you how to apply it to specific behaviors. The techniques may sound tedious, or too simple, or too compulsive, or too difficult, or any number of things, but we have found that approaching these longstanding habits slowly and methodically, a step at a time, works best. These techniques have the historical advantage of working for most people who use them.

This approach to the problem of obesity is quite different from traditional psychotherapy. You probably will not gain insight into the possible psychological reasons for your excess weight, nor will you achieve dramatic solutions to any deep personal problems. That's not the point; the object of these lessons is simply to help you learn new eating skills.

Be on the lookout for a couple of common problems, which you may run into during the program: The tendency to feel or say, "I am fat and will never be able to change"; a "what the hell" attitude, that will clearly defeat you; or, "That's a good idea, but I couldn't possibly do it because . . . ," a self-defeating pattern of rejecting help that will also lead to failure. Weight loss is a matter of arranging priorities in your life. Your eating habits mesh with your social habits, work, recreation, etc. It is hard to change part of the system without an effect on the other parts. Again, one reason we will start slowly in changing behaviors is because it is difficult to change deeply-rooted patterns that interlock with many other behaviors.

The way to learn new habits is through a series of exercises that you can approach creatively. Use that spark of brilliance inside yourself to make it work!

Remember also, the more you can involve others—your family, friends, people at work, or even total strangers—the better your chances of success. Don't be afraid to tell them you are doing something new. If you can get the people around you to help keep track of your behaviors, to help prompt or cue you, it will be much easier to change. This weight control program should be a serious undertaking—your willingness to read this book indicates that kind of commitment. It can be an enjoyable experience, and if taken a step at a time, it is not difficult. Even climbing a mountain like Everest can be broken down into single simple steps taken one at a time. Like mountain climbing, if you try to go too fast or skip steps, you have a greater chance of failing. Habit change is not a race—relax and do it a step at a time.

Pause and Consider What Has Been Covered.

- Do you have any questions about the Food Diary? Yes _____
  No_____

  1. The basic task, instructions, reasons for filling it out, how it works, etc.? (page 10)

  2. The mechanics of filling it out or questions about definitions? (page 13)

- Did you notice any effect of the Food Diary on your eating? Yes_____ No_____ Perhaps_____

- Be sure to fill out the Diary after each meal. Some people carry a pocket notebook, others a 3 x 5 card in their pocket, while others tear out and fold up the Diary pages and carry them around. The immediacy of filling it out, and considering what you have eaten after each meal, is very important. If the papers get greasy or have tomato soup on them, that's O.K.—they're for your use—use them in whatever way helps you.

- From now on, do not include coffee or tea if it has no calories and does not lead to further eating. (The first week you kept track of *all* eating behaviors so you could establish your eating baseline.)

- If you miss a day, that is O.K. Start again the next meal. Filling it out will become more natural with time. Being aware of the food you are eating is one of the strongest of all habits you can develop to limit your food intake. It is possible to extend the concept of a Food Diary ahead in time and use it to plan in advance for snacks and meals. The method for doing this will be presented in a later lesson.

- The Food Diary will change from week to week depending on the topic at hand. We have eliminated some of the columns in the Diary for this week, in order to focus your attention on what we feel to be the vital part of today's lesson.

NEW TOPIC: CUE ELIMINATION—GETTING RID OF THOSE RED FLAGS THAT SIGNAL "TIME TO EAT"

You have probably noticed how walking past a vending machine, a bakery, or a restaurant where you have had several good meals can evoke the feeling of hunger even though you may have recently eaten. Other examples of very strong environmental cues concern place and activity. A person who eats in many different places in his home may eventually experience hunger or the expectation of having something to eat when he is in these places; for example, in the kitchen or living room, or in front of an open refrigerator. One of the most common activity cues for eating is television, where a certain show, like the 6:00 p.m. news, has been paired with eating for a long time and now immediately evokes hunger when it comes on.

In the first lesson you learned that overweight people are more sensitive, and seem to be under a greater degree of situational or stimulus control than non-overweight people. That is, you are more likely than a thin friend to feel hungry when you see or smell food. You are more sensitive to these stimuli. But this sensitivity is not limited to situations or places directly related to foods, such as the smell or sight of something to eat. The environmental cues that stimulate the sensation of hunger can include the time of day, the television set, the telephone, or your car. Any neutral stimulus in the environment, if paired for a long enough time with eating, will acquire the ability to cause the sensation of hunger.

You may have heard of Pavlov's dogs. These animals learned to salivate at the sound of a bell. They did this because they learned to expect food when they heard the experimenter ring his bell. Part of their anticipation of food was salivation. Humans have the same type of reaction to events connected with food. One patient realized, after looking at her Food Diary, that she always felt hungry when she came in the front door of her house. For years she had followed entering the house with a trip to the refrigerator and snacking. She had paired entering the front door with eating for so long that the front door had become a stimulus for hunger. Her hunger, of course, had nothing to do with how physically hungry her body was or how low her blood sugar might have been. It was aroused solely by entering the house through the front door.

Time itself can become the cue to eat. The sensitivity of overweight people to time was shown very vividly in a series of ingenious psychology experiments by Leonard Schacter.[3] He wanted to see if there was any difference between the perceived passage of time and hunger. His basic tool was a pair of peculiar clocks, one of which ran at half normal speed, the other at twice normal speed. The experiments were carried out at 5:00 in the evening, and were presented to the subjects as studies of their personalities and nervous systems. After removing the subject's watch, and attaching wires that went to a machine which supposedly measured nervous activity, the subject was left alone in the room with one of the special clocks on the wall.

In one of the two rooms, the experimenter came back into the room when the slow clock read 5:20; in the other, he came back when the fast clock read 6:05. In each case the real time elapsed was 30 minutes.

When the experimenter entered the room, he was nibbling on crackers from a box. He set the box down in front of the subject, invited him to help himself, and after removing the wires, gave him a personality test (to reinforce the illusion that he was there for a personality test). The subject was left alone to take the test and asked simply to drop it off at the office on his way out of the building. There were two groups of subjects, one normal weight, the other overweight. What was actually measured was the weight of crackers consumed.

Obese subjects ate almost twice as much when they thought the time was 6:05 as they did when they thought that it was 5:20. Thin subjects ate fewer crackers at "6:05," because (they later said) they did not want to spoil their dinners. The study showed that environmental time cues affected the eating of both normal and obese subjects, but in different ways: the belief that dinner time had come stimulated snack eating on the part of the overweight subjects, while it inhibited eating in the thin subjects. The real time of day did not seem to matter. Hunger was controlled by what time the subjects believed it was.

These examples, and this one experiment in particular, show the strong effect environmental cues can have on your life, especially on your eating behaviors.

Try to Apply These Ideas to Yourself.

- Were you aware of how cues signal people to eat or feel hungry?
  Yes_____ No_____

- Try to think of an example of an environmental cue in your life
  that provokes hunger . . . some signal that reminds you to eat
  or snack. These can be at home, at work, while traveling, studying
  —at any time or place or connected with any activity.
  List three: 1. _____

  2. _____

  3. _____

CUE ELIMINATION—HOW TO DO IT!

The techniques of cue elimination will require some cooperation from the
people around you, both at home and at work. Cue related behaviors
are difficult to change, because they often involve other people, especially
at home, and may require some changes in the physical arrangement
of your household.

Last lesson you drew a rough plan of your house and indicated
on it where each eating episode took place. Most people find clusters
of snacks around the television set, by favorite chairs, or in the kitchen
by the refrigerator or sink.

How About You?

- Did you notice any patterns to your eating? Yes_____
  No_____

- Were there more separate eating places than you anticipated?
  Yes_____ No_____

Because you are likely to eat in response to external cues, it makes
sense that eliminating the cues will break up your eating habits. Thus,
if you break the association between T-V and eating, watching T-V will
no longer make you hungry. Similarly, if you do all of your eating in one
place in your house, after a while the other places will no longer remind
you to eat. Eliminating all of the stimuli which evoke feelings of hunger
is difficult, probably impossible in one step. The easiest way to start is
with a set of exercises designed to help you eliminate eating cues; they
make up a six-part assignment as follows:

1. Choose a specific place in one room of your home to do all of your eating. This will be your Designated Appropriate Eating Place. It can be in the kitchen, dining room, or den, and may be different for each meal. It should be a place where you can sit down and eat in relative comfort. From today on, eat all of your meals and snacks at your Designated Appropriate Eating Place. When you have meals away from home, such as work, or when out for a meal, the Designated Appropriate Eating Place will be just that—a place that you consider to be appropriate. This might be a table in a restaurant, cafeteria, or lunchroom.

   When you eat at work, avoid eating at your desk. The object of cue elimination tasks is to break up the association between eating and other activities such as working. If there is no place to eat other than at your desk, at least change it by adding a place mat and silverware and a real cup for your coffee. Try to make it look different from the place where you work. In one experimental situation researchers discovered that a brightly colored place mat helped people designate an eating place which later became a cue for appropriate eating behaviors. For some people a change of this type at work or home is a great help.

   Make your eating place special. From today on eating should be a point of luxury in your life, something to enjoy. Do everything you can to make your eating place pleasant. You can include flowers, music, a comfortable seat, pretty plates, your best silverware—but most important, include enough time. All of these pleasant additions to your eating place will be cues for a new eating style.

2. If your appropriate eating place is the regular dining table, change your habitual eating place at the table. If you sit at the head of the table, change to the side; if you sit on one side, change places with someone on the other side. This may make things a little less efficient for a while, but it also will break up a lot of longstanding cues at the table. This change need not be forever; just to try for a few weeks and see what happens.

3. When eating, only eat. Don't talk on the phone, watch television, read, work, etc. Concentrate on your food and those with you. We want you to really taste your food, feel the textures, and try to enjoy each mouthful—make each meal enjoyable.

4. Remove food from all places in the house other than appropriate storage areas such as the kitchen. Examples are candy on the television set, nuts in the living room, etc. Keep stored food out of sight. This can be done by putting food in cupboards, or keeping it in opaque containers that you cannot see through. Do the same

for foods in the refrigerator—put everything in "see-proof" containers. To further reduce the strength of the visual cues, you can put lower wattage bulbs in the kitchen area where you prepare and store food, and replace your refrigerator light with a dim one—or remove it altogether.

5. Have other foods on hand to replace junk or convenience foods—if you must have both in the house, keep one, the healthy one, visible in an attractive container, the empty-calorie food out of sight in a dark container. It will help you decide which to eat when the impulse to snack comes along.

6. Do not keep serving containers on the table while you eat. If this is not possible, put the serving dishes at the other end of the table from where you sit.

The behavior changes introduced in this lesson are difficult to master. Eating in one place is difficult at first for many people. Remember to eat only in a place that you designate as appropriate. The object of this exercise is to eliminate cues that you have traditionally associated with food; with time and lack of use, these cues will return to a neutral state where food is concerned. Your new eating place will take over this cueing function and it will begin to remind you of a new set of eating behaviors.

You probably will not be able to accomplish these cue elimination exercises immediately, even though they sound very simple. They are not simple for everyone. If you are not completely successful the first week, do not feel guilty or give up; try to do a little better each day.

One way to improve your chances of success is to provide yourself with some form of information about your progress. Among the homework forms you will find a type of graph, a scatter diagram entitled "Eating Place Record," to help you keep track of how much you are improving each day. Start filling it in today, at the start of Week Two. You will use it for the next three weeks.

You will find seven common eating places listed under "Place" on the Eating Place Record, and one additional line labeled "Other." Use this line if you eat at places not on the list. The "Designated Eating Place" will be the place that you have chosen for your meals and snacks. Almost always it will include a table and chair, and it usually will be the same place at least for the same meal each day; for example, the kitchen table for breakfast, a table at the cafeteria at work for lunch, and at the dining room table for dinner. You can include restaurants, lunch rooms, picnics—any place that you feel is appropriate for meals away from home. If you have a snack, take it to the place you have designated as appropriate before you eat it.

There are six numbers under each day of the week on the Eating Place Record. These refer to consecutive eating episodes—snacks or meals. Each day, check the box that indicates where each eating episode took place. The ideal is a straight line with the "Designated Eating Place" checked for every meal or snack. The closer you can come to this ideal (as shown in the completed sample), the closer you will come to eliminating a large number of environmental cues that may be reminding you to eat, or may be making you momentarily hungry when you really aren't. Again, you will be most successful with cue elimination if you get help from your family and friends. Tell them what you are doing and the reasons for it. You will find that explaining the techniques to others will help you understand them better yourself. Your family's enthusiasm can only help.

Many other cues can be eliminated from your immediate environment—all of the little signals that say "eat": leftovers, snacks, vending machines, shopping, etc. A technique can be devised for each of these to eliminate specific causes of impulse eating, and they will be discussed later. However, this week concentrate on the six exercises introduced above.

The final column on the Food Diary for this lesson is labeled, "Food out of sight." Put a check mark in this column if food was in containers and out of sight before the meal or snack, and if serving containers were not prominent on the table during meals. (Again, if they cannot be taken off the table, arrange for them to be as far away from you as possible—to reduce their effectiveness as a cue.)

In summary, this week start eliminating cues from your environment that might be triggers for hungry feelings. Food should assume a low profile in your home. The keys to this are: eating in one place; changing your eating place at the table; only eating at mealtimes; removing food from storage areas; having foods on hand to replace junk foods; and removing serving dishes from the table.

HOMEWORK.

    A. Lesson Two Food Diary.

    B. Eating Place Record filled in for each meal and snack during the coming week.

    C. Designate an appropriate eating place at home and work. Eat all of your meals and snacks at this place.

    D. Change your habitual eating place at the table.

    E. When eating, only eat. No other activities.

    F. Remove food from all places in the house which are not appropriate storage areas. Reduce visual cues for eating. Store food in opaque containers.

G. Keep junk foods out of sight, hidden, hard to get, or don't buy them.

H. Remove serving dishes from the table or put them at the opposite end of the table.

Mark the last column of the Food Diary "yes" or "no" to indicate whether visual cues were reduced for each meal or snack. Remember, if you are going to eat, make it worthwhile.

FOOD DIARY – Lesson Two

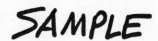

Day of Week __MONDAY__   Name ___C.B.T.___

Time	Minutes Spent Eating	M/S	H	Activity While Eating	Location of Eating	Type & Quantity of Food	Food Out of Sight
6:00							
7:20 – 7:30	10 MIN	M	0	PAPER	KITCHEN	COFFEE, CEREAL	✓
8:15 – 8:20	5 MIN	S	0	TALKING	WORK	COFFEE, DONUT	
11:00							
3:30 – 3:40	10 MIN	M	3	READING	RESTAUR.	HAMBURG.	✓
4:00							
6:00 – 7:00	1 HR	M	2	TV	DR.	BEEF TV DINNER ICE CREAM	✓
9:00							
10:30 – 10:45	15 MIN	S	0	TV	LR	ICE CREAM	✓

M/S – Meal or Snack
H – Hunger (0 = None; 3 = Maximum)

FOOD DIARY – Lesson Two

Day of Week _____   Name _____

Time	Minutes Spent Eating	M/S	H	Activity While Eating	Location of Eating	Type & Quantity of Food	Food Out of Sight
6:00							
11:00							
4:00							
9:00							

M/S – Meal or Snack
H – Hunger (0 = None; 3 = Maximum)

FOOD DIARY – Lesson Two

Day of Week _____   Name _____

Time	Minutes Spent Eating	M/S	H	Activity While Eating	Location of Eating	Type & Quantity of Food	Food Out of Sight
6:00							
11:00							
4:00							
9:00							

M/S – Meal or Snack
H – Hunger (0 = None; 3 = Maximum)

FOOD DIARY – Lesson Two

Day of Week _____   Name _____

Time	Minutes Spent Eating	M/S	H	Activity While Eating	Location of Eating	Type & Quantity of Food	Food Out of Sight
6:00							
11:00							
4:00							
9:00							

M/S – Meal or Snack
H – Hunger (0 = None; 3 = Maximum)

FOOD DIARY – Lesson Two

Day of Week _____   Name_____

Time	Minutes Spent Eating	M/S	H	Activity While Eating	Location of Eating	Type & Quantity of Food	Food Out of Sight
6:00							
11:00							
4:00							
9:00							

M/S – Meal or Snack
H – Hunger (0 = None; 3 = Maximum)

FOOD DIARY – Lesson Two

Day of Week _____   Name _____

Time	Minutes Spent Eating	M/S	H	Activity While Eating	Location of Eating	Type & Quantity of Food	Food Out of Sight
6:00							
11:00							
4:00							
9:00							

M/S – Meal or Snack
H – Hunger (0 = None; 3 = Maximum)

FOOD DIARY – Lesson Two

Day of Week _____   Name_____

Time	Minutes Spent Eating	M/S	H	Activity While Eating	Location of Eating	Type & Quantity of Food	Food Out of Sight
6:00							
11:00							
4:00							
9:00							

M/S – Meal or Snack
H – Hunger (0 = None; 3 = Maximum)

FOOD DIARY – Lesson Two

Day of Week _____   Name _____

Time	Minutes Spent Eating	M/S	H	Activity While Eating	Location of Eating	Type & Quantity of Food	Food Out of Sight
6:00							
11:00							
4:00							
9:00							

M/S – Meal or Snack
H – Hunger (0 = None; 3 = Maximum)

SAMPLE

EATING PLACE RECORD

Name _____

(Numbers under the days of the week refer to consecutive eating episodes)

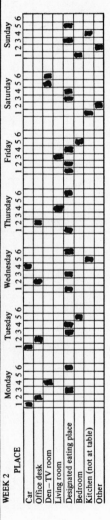

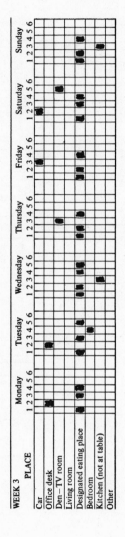

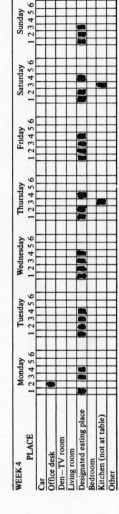

EATING PLACE RECORD

Name _____

(Numbers under the days of the week refer to consecutive eating episodes)

WEEK 2

PLACE	Monday 1 2 3 4 5 6	Tuesday 1 2 3 4 5 6	Wednesday 1 2 3 4 5 6	Thursday 1 2 3 4 5 6	Friday 1 2 3 4 5 6	Saturday 1 2 3 4 5 6	Sunday 1 2 3 4 5 6
Car							
Office desk							
Den—TV room							
Living room							
Designated eating place							
Bedroom							
Kitchen (not at table)							
Other							

WEEK 3

PLACE	Monday 1 2 3 4 5 6	Tuesday 1 2 3 4 5 6	Wednesday 1 2 3 4 5 6	Thursday 1 2 3 4 5 6	Friday 1 2 3 4 5 6	Saturday 1 2 3 4 5 6	Sunday 1 2 3 4 5 6
Car							
Office desk							
Den—TV room							
Living room							
Designated eating place							
Bedroom							
Kitchen (not at table)							
Other							

WEEK 4

PLACE	Monday 1 2 3 4 5 6	Tuesday 1 2 3 4 5 6	Wednesday 1 2 3 4 5 6	Thursday 1 2 3 4 5 6	Friday 1 2 3 4 5 6	Saturday 1 2 3 4 5 6	Sunday 1 2 3 4 5 6
Car							
Office desk							
Den—TV room							
Living room							
Designated eating place							
Bedroom							
Kitchen (not at table)							
Other							

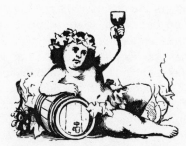

Lesson Three

Changing the Act of Eating

WEIGH-IN AND HOMEWORK.

Weigh yourself and record your weight. Calculate and plot your weight change on your Master Data Sheet. (The average weight change for an individual at this point in this program is roughly two pounds. This is shown by the diagonal line across the graph on your Master Data Sheet.)

Check your homework for Lesson Two and Record whether or not you completed it on the Homework Credit Sheet.

—Is your Lesson Two Food Diary complete? Yes_____ No_____

—Is the "Food out of sight" column in the Food Diary checked for every day? Yes_____ No_____

—Is your Eating Place Record filled in for this week? Yes_____ No_____

REVIEW.

Last week's lesson reviewed the theory of behavior modification and the concept of over-eating as a learned behavior. Since eating behaviors are learned, the logical way to change them is to learn competing or opposing behaviors, or to change the environment in a way which will eliminate the associated behavior. The effect on the original habits is that without practice they become weaker, and eventually are extinguished. It is very important to *be consistent.* If you practice not eating in front of the television set for three weeks, and then start again, you will very rapidly reestablish your old association of television with food, and television may re-emerge as an even stronger environmental cue than before.

Last week much of the discussion concerned the effect of environmental cues on eating behaviors. Many kinds of cues were identified: place cues, activity cues, time cues, etc. Any stimulus paired long enough with eating will signal you to feel hunger, or to want to be fed when you encounter it. The technique of cue elimination was introduced as a systematic way of breaking up these patterns of cue and response. If you no longer eat after you open the refrigerator, the refrigerator will, with time, lose the hunger-provoking quality it may have now.

You drew a House Plan and marked on it every place where you had either a meal or a snack. The object of this exercise was to give you a graphic representation of where you eat, and a way of analyzing what the surrounding cues are. Most people find they eat in different places throughout the house, and some are able to see from the House Plan which cues are telling them to eat.

Several exercises in cue elimination were introduced, designed to break up the associations between eating cues and eating responses at home.

1. The technique most emphasized last week was choosing a specific place (or if necessary, more than one) for your eating, your *Designated Appropriate Eating Place,* and eating all of your meals and snacks there. For meals eaten out of the house, for example, at work, such a place might have to be a restaurant, or some other place you feel is appropriate. This is a behavior change that is difficult, because it is a major change and involves other members of the family.

    You filled in a scatter diagram Eating Place Record to help you with this change. The object of the diagram was to give you immediate feedback about the location of your meals and snacks, and to make you demonstrate to yourself how close to ideal you were in your behavior as you approached a straight line on the diagram.

Let's Consider the Eating
Place Record for a Moment

- Did you understand how to fill it out? Yes_____ No_____
(Pages 32, 33)

- Did you achieve a straight line on the diagram? Yes_____
No_____

- Did you notice any effect of this technique on the amount you ate last week?

2. You were asked to *change places with someone at the table* to see how different the meals look from another vantage point. A side effect of this technique is to make you extra aware of mealtime, of the changes that are going on in your eating habits, and to provide the social setting for change. Everyone at the table will be aware of your change, and this can give you a starting point for eating differently.

How Did This Work Out?

- Did you experience any difference changing from your customary eating place? Yes_____ No_____

- Any comment from your family? Yes_____ No_____

- Was it helpful? Yes_____ No_____

- What did you do to make your eating place special?

   1. _____

   2. _____

3. You were to *eat only during meals,* avoiding any associated activity not appropriate to enjoying a good meal. You were to concentrate on your food, to try to be a gourmet, to taste and try to enjoy every mouthful. The reason for this was to break up associations between activities like reading a paper in the mid-morning and hunger. When you are hungry, only eat.

How Did This Go?

- Did you pay more attention to your meals as a result of this technique? Yes_____ No_____

- Do you remember why this is such an important exercise? Yes_____ No_____

It is very important that you continue applying this technique. It becomes easier with time. You will find meals will be more enjoyable, food tastier, and conversation more lively without the television. Doing without diversions is difficult at first, but it gets easier.

4. Next, you were to *remove all food from non-storage places* in the house; for example, by the bed or on top of the television set. The reason for this was to remove the cue of food itself from your home environment. This should have been easy, because you located all of your eating places on your House Plan last week.

In addition to putting food in proper storage areas, you were to make food less visible. Some of the techniques suggested were putting food in opaque containers, putting dim bulbs in food preparation areas, and putting a smaller light in your refrigerator (or taking it out altogether). All of these tactics help you counteract the hunger cues built into the sight of food. When food is stored conspicuously, it looks and smells more appealing and it makes you hungry. When it is out of sight, it no longer has that power. You were asked to keep track in your Food Diary of attempts to keep food out of sight.

Was There Any Trouble?

- This technique often involves the family, and sometimes it requires their cooperation to get the potato chips out of the den. Did you encounter any family resistance? Yes_____ No_____
- Will it be difficult to continue keeping food in the proper storage places? Yes_____ No_____
- Did you put your food in opaque ("see-proof") containers? Yes_____ No_____
- Did you go all the way and take the bulb out of your refrigerator? Yes_____ No_____

5. You were urged to keep alternate low-calorie foods on hand if necessary for the sudden urges to eat. *High-impulse or junk foods* should either not be purchased or kept in a place where they cannot reach out and grab your appetite; for example, in a dark container or, if appropriate, in the freezer.

Did you put the junk foods out of sight? Yes____No____

6. Another technique to decrease impulse eating is to *remove serving dishes from the table.* If this proved impossible, you were to place them at the end of the table farthest away from you, to minimize their effect on your eating.

Was This Helpful?

- Were you able to do this? Yes_____ No_____
- Did your family object to this technique? Yes_____ No_____

If you haven't been able to use all of these techniques in one week, don't worry; it is not a setback. Everyone goes at his or her own pace. More time may be needed to change what for you might be a more difficult or stronger habit than for someone else. Take another week and work on them, until you feel satisfied that they are mastered—then go on.

Be creative in your solutions. There are many ways to go about cue elimination. When you become aware of eating in response to a cue in your environment, any place or any time, try to disassociate it from eating and food.

We will keep referring to a particular point in connection with all of the changes in behaviors we make in this course: the important concept of "Maintenance." If you don't keep track of new behaviors, they fade away with time. In a few weeks we will introduce a checklist for new behaviors, so you can monitor yourself and insure that your new behaviors are continuing. This mechanical checking can be reduced or eliminated with time, but while the changes are fresh, we will ask you to check your behaviors daily, then eventually to change to weekly or monthly self-evaluation. For the next week though, keep working on the cue elimination assignments and filling in the Eating Place Record, in addition to the weekly Food Diary.

NEW TECHNIQUE: CHANGING THE ACT OF EATING.

The behavior you will work on this week is the actual act of eating. Many people who are overweight have a habit of eating without pause, as much food as fast as possible. If you compared the bites per minute of an overweight person with those of a normal-weight person, you would find that thin people eat fast at first, but soon slow down. People who are overweight tend to keep eating rapidly throughout the meal. Eating fast, without pausing or slowing down, is a bad habit. It leads to excessive eating. It takes time for the food you eat to be absorbed into your system and decrease your hunger. There is a better chance of becoming satiated, of feeling full, and a much better chance of enjoying your meal, if you slow down—take thirty minutes instead of five. By slowing down your rate of eating you may find a dramatic change in how you eat, and you will feel no more hungry than when you ate more.

Telling you to eat more slowly may be helpful, but introducing specific techniques to help you eat more slowly is a better way to approach the problem. Most people have the habit of placing more food on their forks while they are still chewing the previous forkful. As soon as they swallow their food they place more food in their mouths, and refill their forks. If you can learn to swallow the food in your mouth before adding more to your fork, you will automatically extend the length of time a meal takes and allow yourself more time to enjoy food.

The long-term goal of this week's assignment is to swallow the food from each bite before any more is added to your eating utensils. The best way to do this, and systematically to change your eating pattern, is to put your utensils down after each bite, and not pick them up until the bite has been swallowed. In the case of handheld food such as a hamburger, put the food down between bites, in the same way you would put down a fork or spoon.

Like eating in one place, if putting your utensils down after each bite is not already a habit, establishing the behavior pattern may be difficult. At first it will feel awkward, uncomfortable, and you will tend to forget.

There are two ways of establishing the habit of putting utensils down between bites: first, simply to do it, and secondly, to work up to it gradually. If you must work up to this behavior gradually, start by observing how frequently you currently put your eating tools down, and then try to increase the frequency. If you find that you can put your fork down once every four bites now, work toward doing it once every two bites, and eventually after each bite.

The best form of feedback on progress in this technique is to record simple ratios: 1:8, 1:4, 1:1, etc. Record the ratio of putting utensils down, to bites, in the last column in your Food Diary this coming week, and see if you can make the 1:1 ratio a habit. To determine what your ratio is, count your bites for five minutes, and at the same time keep track of the number of times you put your fork or spoon down. For example, 50 bites with the utensils put down ten times would be a ratio of 10:50, or 1:5.

Either do the counting yourself, or have someone around you count for you during the first five minutes of your meals. This technique is like eating in one place, or only eating while eating. It sounds simple, but can be very difficult when you try to do it.

You must plan to take some time to change your old habits and to introduce new ones. Be creative in your approach. One person bought himself a place setting of stainless steel utensils. He found that if he set his place with this new knife, fork, and spoon rather than his usual ones, he automatically remembered to eat differently, to slow down, and to put the utensils down between bites. The unfamiliar feel of the new eating utensils reminded him to use his new eating habits. Another cue that can help is the use of special plates or place mats, or anything to make your eating place special. To help you keep track of your bite-fork ratio, it often helps to have a card that says "count," or a block or pyramid with different ratio numbers on different sides on the table with the appropriate side turned toward you.

If you are already successfully putting your fork down after each bite, if you have found it easy to do so, jump ahead and try an additional delaying technique: After you can swallow each bite, and before you put more food on your fork, introduce a two-minute delay at some point in your meal. This can be either after a pre-set number of minutes, or after a specific course. Take the two minutes to talk, to relax, and to enjoy the meal. However, as long as you have trouble putting down your utensils between bites, concentrate only on that. It can be a difficult eating pattern to develop, and it should be practiced exclusively until it becomes habit.

Once again, be creative! There are many ways to stretch out a meal. Try to use as many delaying techniques as possible. Eating should be pleasurable. You should have time to taste, to chew, to experience all of the food you eat. Practice being more of a gourmet. Relax, slow down, and enjoy your food by concentrating on its taste, texture, sight, and smell.

Do You Feel Comfortable About This New Technique?

- Do you have any questions about the reason for putting your eating utensils down between bites? Yes_____ No_____ (If yes, reread this section.)

- Do you understand how to do it? Yes_____ No_____ (Pages 50, 51)

- If you already put your utensils down between bites (always), what is your next step? (Answer: to swallow between bites with your utensil on the table, and then to put in a two-minute delay in mid-meal.)

HOMEWORK.

A. Lesson Three Food Diary.

B. Fill in the eating ratio column on the Lesson Three Food Diary.

C. Continue to fill in the Eating Place Record every day.

D. Continue to carry out the cue elimination exercises:

1. Eat all of your meals and snacks in a Designated Appropriate Eating Place.

2. Change places at the table.

3. When you eat, only eat. No other activities.

4. Eliminate visual cues. Remove food from inappropriate or non-storage areas in the house. Make food inconspicuous—put it in opaque containers.

5. Keep alternate foods available to help keep from snacking on "junk" foods.

6. Remove serving dishes from the table, or put them as far away as possible from you on the table.

FOOD DIARY – Lesson Three

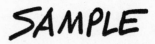

Day of Week _MONDAY_   Name _C. B. T._

Time	Minutes Spent Eating	M/S	H	Activity While Eating	Location of Eating	Food Type & Quantity	Eating Ratio
6:00							
7:20-7:30	10 MIN	M	0	PAPER	KITCHEN	COFFEE, CEREAL	1:8
8:15 - 8:20	5 MIN	S	0	TALKING	WORK	COFFEE, DONUT	1:8
11:00							
3:30 - 3:40	10 MIN	M	3	READING	RESTAUR.	HAMBURG.	1:4
4:00							
6:00-7:00	1 HR	M	2	TV	DR.	BEEF TV DINNER ICE CREAM	1:1
9:00							
10:30-10:45	15 MIN	S	0	TV	LR	ICE CREAM	1:2

FOOD DIARY – **Lesson Three**

Day of Week _____   Name _____

Time	Minutes Spent Eating	M/S	H	Activity While Eating	Location of Eating	Food Type & Quantity	Eating Ratio
6:00							
11:00							
4:00							
9:00							

FOOD DIARY – Lesson Three

Day of Week _____   Name_____

Time	Minutes Spent Eating	M/S	H	Activity While Eating	Location of Eating	Food Type & Quantity	Eating Ratio
6:00							
11:00							
4:00							
9:00							

FOOD DIARY -- Lesson Three

Day of Week _____   Name _____

Time	Minutes Spent Eating	M/S	H	Activity While Eating	Location of Eating	Food Type & Quantity	Eating Ratio
6:00							
11:00							
4:00							
9:00							

FOOD DIARY – Lesson Three

Day of Week _____   Name_____

Time	Minutes Spent Eating	M/S	H	Activity While Eating	Location of Eating	Food Type & Quantity	Eating Ratio
6:00							
11:00							
4:00							
9:00							

FOOD DIARY – Lesson Three

Day of Week _____   Name_____

Time	Minutes Spent Eating	M/S	H	Activity While Eating	Location of Eating	Food Type & Quantity	Eating Ratio
6:00							
11:00							
4:00							
9:00							

FOOD DIARY – **Lesson Three**

Day of Week _____   Name_____

Time	Minutes Spent Eating	M/S	H	Activity While Eating	Location of Eating	Food Type & Quantity	Eating Ratio
6:00							
11:00							
4:00							
9:00							

FOOD DIARY – Lesson Three

Day of Week _____   Name _____

Time	Minutes Spent Eating	M/S	H	Activity While Eating	Location of Eating	Food Type & Quantity	Eating Ratio
6:00							
11:00							
4:00							
9:00							

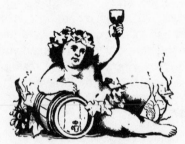

Lesson Four

Behavior Chains and Alternate Activities

WEIGH-IN AND HOMEWORK.

Weigh yourself and fill in your Master Data Sheet.

The cumulative average weight loss for group treatment at Lesson Four has been about three pounds. Graph your weekly weight loss and compare it with the "average" represented by the diagonal line on the Master Data Sheet.

Check Your Homework.

—Is your Lesson Three Food Diary complete? Yes_____ No_____

—Has the Eating Ratio column been completely filled in? Yes_____ No_____

—Is your Eating Place Record up to date? Yes_____
No_____

Give yourself credit towards your refund on your Homework Credit
Sheet.

REVIEW.

This program stresses eating behaviors rather than nutrition, calories, or
the emotions associated with eating. Although there has been no discussion of *self-observation* as such, actually it has been your prime method
of assessing eating behaviors. You have kept meticulous track of your
food intake, the time, place, and reasons for eating, in addition to records
of the type of food you eat. This recording has sensitized you to your
eating behaviors and has made you very aware of your food intake. The
Food Diary has been the principal tool in helping you change your percep-
tion of food. It can be a very powerful aid in reshaping your eating habits
and maintaining these habits once they have been established.

How Are You Doing?

- Are you keeping track of your food intake on the Food Diary forms?
  Yes_____ No_____

- Are you having difficulty filling out the Diary? Yes_____
  No_____ (See Page 13)

- Are you giving yourself credit for completed homework?
  Yes_____ No_____

- Many people can see emerging patterns of eating behaviors, and
  changes in their eating habits by this point in the program—can
  you? Yes_____ No_____

During the second lesson you learned that overweight people are
more sensitive than thin people to environmental stimuli, to those little
reminders around you that signal "Eat." These stimuli, or cues, include
places, times, events, emotions, social situations, etc. Any object, feeling
or place can become a reminder to eat, and can evoke hunger if it is
paired with food for a long enough period of time. Some examples given
were television programs, the refrigerator, and, in one case, the front door.

The homework assignment for that week had six parts, each designed to disconnect a set of cue-related eating patterns. These were:

1. Choosing a Designated Appropriate Eating Place.

2. Switching places at the table.

3. Doing nothing else when eating.

4. Making food less visible by storing it in opaque containers, and removing food from other areas in the house.

5. Minimizing the attraction of "junk"—or "empty-calorie" foods.

6. Taking serving dishes off the table.

Choosing the Designated Appropriate Eating Place was emphasized particularly, because it is often the most useful in breaking habits. We provided you with an Eating Place Record or scatter diagram, to keep track of where your meals and snacks were eaten. It is a tool to help you change. A straight line on it indicates you were at your designated place every time you had something to eat.

How Do You Feel About That Assignment?

- Was there any difficulty continuing with the assignment the second week? Yes_____ No_____

- Do you understand what this homework assignment was supposed to accomplish? Yes_____ No_____ (Page 49)

- Is it becoming easier to eat in only one place? Yes_____ No_____

It is important to practice all of the cue elimination exercises every time you have something to eat. Check the following to see how well you are doing:

	Yes	No
A. Are you storing food in opaque containers?	_____	_____
B. Did you acquire special "see-proof" containers for food?	_____	_____
C. Is food more out of sight at home now than before?	_____	_____
D. Is junk food either not purchased or kept out of sight?	_____	_____
E. Are you doing nothing else when you eat?	_____	_____

F. What are some of your remaining cues for eating, and what can be done to eliminate them?

1. _____

2. _____

In the coming months, you will find the strength of old environmental cues diminishing. Many people report that 12 to 15 weeks of cue elimination practice are necessary to return strong cues, like television, to neutral. At that point the cue no longer makes them hungry and does not remind them of food.

Lesson Three discussed the fact that overweight people tend to eat faster and more continuously than thin people. You were asked to interrupt this tendency by adding a behavior that forced you to eat more slowly: putting your fork down between bites. The method of observation you used was either self-report (you counted your bites and the number of times you put your utensils down), or someone else counted for you. A ratio of forkfuls to swallows was suggested as a way of keeping track of how well you were adopting this new habit.

The final point of the last lesson was positive "cueing." One of the most difficult parts of the entire program is cueing (building reminders of the assigned behaviors into your environment). A card on the table, a reminder from your spouse, or a block or pyramid with numbers painted on it can be a very useful reminder of your desired eating ratio for that meal.

How Did You Do With This Technique?

- Did you have any problems with the idea or with the mechanics of eating slowly? Yes_____ No_____

- Do you understand why it is a useful technique? Yes_____ No_____ (Page 50)

- My eating ratio today was _____ : _____.

Slow eating is a habit you should continue to practice. For the next few weeks continue eating slowly and continue to record your eating ratio in the last column of the Food Diary.

A second technique was introduced for those who had mastered putting their utensils down after each bite. This was to swallow food between bites and to put a time delay of two minutes into the meal, either at a pre-set time or after a certain course (like salad). During this time you are simply to sit and talk, think pleasant thoughts, listen to the radio, or leave the table and do some alternate activity. This delay will allow time to pass, and the time will enable your brain to sense that your stomach has been fed.

Has This Been Effective?

- Did you try this technique? Yes_____ No_____

- Do you see how it could be a useful technique? Yes_____ No_____ (Page 51)

NEW TECHNIQUE: BEHAVIOR
CHAINS AND ALTERNATE ACTIVITIES.

Using activities to break up patterns of behaviors that lead to inappropriate eating can be a very powerful means of changing eating habits. Activity substitution is a technique that is particularly useful when you are eating in response to environmental as well as internal cues. These can include the hunger pangs you feel at odd times; for example, after meals, before bed, or when you are out shopping.

The principle behind activity substitution is quite simple. Behaviors occur in chains. Eating (or more precisely, feeling bad about eating) is at one end of a chain of responses. As you work backwards from the terminal behaviors, you can recognize events or cues in your environment that started the chain of events that led to eating. For example:

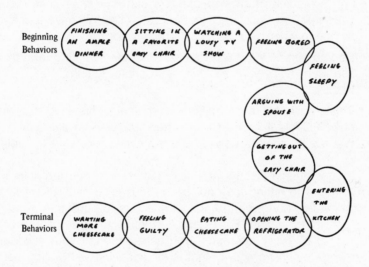

If the chain is broken at any point, it probably will not continue, and the final behaviors in the chain, eating and feeling guilty, will not occur. The earlier in the chain you identify the trend towards eating, the easier it is to intervene. If you don't identify the chain until you have opened the refrigerator door, it may be too late.

The interventions can be very simple. Once the behavior chain has been identified, it is a matter of selecting an alternative activity that will either not progress toward eating, or will delay eating until your hunger has diminished.

In the above example, you may recognize that your favorite chair always leads to this chain of behaviors after dinner. Watching T-V somewhere else may break the chain. A more stimulating T-V show, or a copy of a sexy book, may keep your attention and break the chain. If you feel sleepy, a ten-minute nap may unlink the chain. A prior agreement with yourself to wash the dishes before having a snack might either save you from the dishwashing chore, or delay your eating until you are no longer hungry. If you got as far as the refrigerator, you could have a pre-prepared alternate snack of carrots or fruit to deter you from the left-over cheesecake.

Finally, if you do eat the cheesecake, try not to feel guilty; you simply were not prepared to break the chain at this time.

Let's Consider This New Concept a Bit.

- Do you understand the concept of behavior chains? Yes_____ No_____ (It is important that you do understand it. Re-read the last section if it is not absolutely clear.)

- Can you think of an example of a behavior chain that occurs in your life? Yes_____ No_____ (You will have a chance to fill one in when you do today's homework.)

- Do you see how breaking a chain like the sample one in this lesson can help you avoid inappropriate eating? Yes_____ No_____

- What would be the easiest link for you to break in this type of chain? Circle it and draw in a new link with an alternate activity that would steer you away from the eating you want to avoid.

If your hunger occurs at a fixed time each day, the links in the chain that lead to eating may not be obvious. The most direct strategy to overcome this hunger and habitual snack is to substitute a non-food related activity for eating. For example, if you know you have a craving for food at 3:15 every afternoon, you can rearrange your schedule so you are engaged in an activity that is incompatible with eating between 2:45 and 3:45. You will be changing the terminal end of the behavior chain by substituting some other activity for your usual 3:15 snack. Alternate activities could include walking the dog, playing tennis, taking a bath, washing your hair, or sleeping. *Hunger pangs are short-lived,* and if you delay eating by 10 or 15 minutes, the urge to eat will usually diminish. The hunger you feel at odd times is probably a conditioned response to a cue in your environment, even though you are not able to identify it while you are responding to it. If feeling hungry is not rewarded with food, the hunger response will diminish with time. The unknown environmental cue will lose its ability to evoke your hunger.

All substitute activities must possess two important qualities: they must be readily available, and they must be able to compete with the urge to eat. Two types of activities can compete with hunger: (a) pleasant activities, and (b) necessary activities—things you have to do each day, hungry or not. Some examples of pleasant substitutions are: a hobby, a walk around the block, working in the garden, reading a good book, listening to music, taking a leisurely bath, and sleeping. Some examples of the necessary type of activities are: errands, cleaning the house, doing homework, working on household projects, making phone calls, paying bills, washing the floor, and washing your hair. If possible the activity you choose should be incompatible with eating.

Consider All of This for a Moment.

- Do you understand what an alternate activity is? Yes_____
  No_____

- Write down a pleasant activity that might be substituted for eating.

  _____

- Write down a necessary activity that could be substituted for eating.

  _____

- Write down an activity that is incompatible with eating. (It may be one of the activities you thought of under "B" or "C.")

  _____

Remember, you are often trying to outwit a hunger pang that has a life expectancy of only 10 to 15 minutes.

A more neutral way to break a behavior chain, especially if you are aware of only the terminal behaviors, is to add time between the links. This is easily accomplished by setting a cooking timer, parking meter, alarm clock, etc. for a pre-set number of minutes, and delaying the snack. At first, interpose one or two minutes. Gradually increase the time between the urge to snack and your actual eating to 10 to 15 minutes. While you are waiting to eat, do something else. You will be amazed at how few snacks you will want if you wait a few minutes between the time you first recognize an urge to eat and the point when you actually open the refrigerator door.

HOMEWORK.

Identify at least one of your eating behavior chains. The homework forms include an Alternate Activity Sheet, which contains a blank chain. Start analyzing your behavior by selecting an eating situation that occurs fairly often during the week. This could be an afternoon snack, an urge for food in the morning, or a bite to eat while watching T-V or studying in the evening. Write down the terminal end, the eating response, and try to fill in each step that precedes it. When you are done, it should look like our earlier example.

After you have defined a behavior chain, plan several alternate activities to break the chain at its weakest links. During the week record whether or not your chain-breaking strategies were successful.

If you can identify only the terminal link in a behavior chain, plan an alternate activity that will take the place of the eating response, or introduce a delay before you eat. The easiest way to make this technique work is to have a list of alternate activities prepared in advance, and introduce them between the urge to snack and the actual eating. On the Alternate Activity Sheet you will find a place to record six alternate responses; three should be activities that are pleasant, that can compete with hunger by being enjoyable, and three should be necessary activities that can compete because you are obligated to do them during the day.

Try to make a substitution every day. Write down each time you are successful in substituting an alternate response for eating.

One strategy that may be useful is to give yourself permission to snack at first, by saying to yourself something like, "I am hungry and I want a snack, but before I eat it, I will_____."

A great deal of extra eating takes place when people are bored or fatigued. If you can prevent boredom, you may be able to prevent over-eating. Your Alternate Activity Sheet may be able to help you do this, by providing an easily accessible list of things to do when you are bored and can't think of anything to do. If you find you are eating because of fatigue, then the appropriate response is a ten-minute nap rather than food. Sometimes it is hard to distinguish between boredom and fatigue—but a nap is not only non-caloric and incompatible with eating, it is also refreshing.

The homework assignment for this week is complicated:

A. Keep up your Lesson Four Food Diary.

B. Continue to fill in the Eating Ratio every day. Try to make it 1:1.

C. Complete the Eating Place Record. This is the third and final week for this form.

D. Fill in the spaces on your Alternate Activity Sheet labeled "Substitute Activity."

E. Write down one of your behavior chains on the Alternate Activity Sheet. Take a few minutes and think it over. Perhaps you will want to discuss it with your family. Regular chains of behaviors occur in all lives—we simply don't pay attention to them.

F. Plan an "unlinking strategy." Find the weak link in your eating behavior chain and plan an alternate activity to hook onto that weak link.

G. Keep track of the situations where you were able to break your eating chain.

FOOD DIARY – Lesson Four

Day of Week_____   Name_____

Time	Min Spent Eating	M/S	H	Body Position	Activity While Eating	Location of Eating	Food Type and Quantity	Ratio
6:00								
11:00								
4:00								
9:00								

FOOD DIARY – Lesson Four

Day of Week_____   Name _____

Time	Min Spent Eating	M/S	H	Body Position	Activity While Eating	Location of Eating	Food Type and Quantity	Ratio
6:00								
11:00								
4:00								
9:00								

FOOD DIARY – Lesson Four

Day of Week_____   Name _____

Time	Min Spent Eating	M/S	H	Body Position	Activity While Eating	Location of Eating	Food Type and Quantity	Ratio
6:00								
11:00								
4:00								
9:00								

FOOD DIARY – Lesson Four

Day of Week_____   Name _____

Time	Min Spent Eating	M/S	H	Body Position	Activity While Eating	Location of Eating	Food Type and Quantity	Ratio
6:00								
11:00								
4:00								
9:00								

FOOD DIARY – Lesson Four

Day of Week_____   Name_____

Time	Min Spent Eating	M/S	H	Body Position	Activity While Eating	Location of Eating	Food Type and Quantity	Ratio
6:00								
11:00								
4:00								
9:00								

FOOD DIARY – Lesson Four

Day of Week_____   Name_____

Time	Min Spent Eating	M/S	H	Body Position	Activity While Eating	Location of Eating	Food Type and Quantity	Ratio
6:00								
11:00								
4:00								
9:00								

FOOD DIARY – Lesson Four

Day of Week_____   Name_____

Time	Min Spent Eating	M/S	H	Body Position	Activity While Eating	Location of Eating	Food Type and Quantity	Ratio
6:00								
11:00								
4:00								
9:00								

ALTERNATE ACTIVITY SHEET

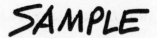

SUBSTITUTE ACTIVITIES

Pleasant Activities   1. _SINGING ~ WASHING HAIR_

                        2. _PLAYING PIANO ~ BIKING_

                        3. _SEWING ~ CALLING "SHUT-INS"_

Necessary Activities   1. _DUSTING_

                        2. _VACUMMING_

                        3. _STRAIGHTEN HOUSE_

Situations when used   1. _WANTED ICE CREAM ~ DELAYED WITH BATH_

                        2. _WANTED WHEAT THINS ~ CLEANED UP YARD_

                        3. _WANTED SNACK ~ WENT FOR WALK_

                        4. _WANTED COOKIES ~ DID DISHES FIRST_

                        5. _SAW LEFT OVERS ~ THREW THEM OUT, WENT FOR BIKE RIDE_

                        6. _TEMPTED BY COOKIES ~ SET TIMER_

                        7. _WANTED SNACK ~ PLAYED PIANO_

BEHAVIOR CHAIN

Identify the links in your eating response chain on the following diagram. Draw a line
through the chain where it was interrupted. Add the link you substituted and the new
chain of behaviors this substitution started.

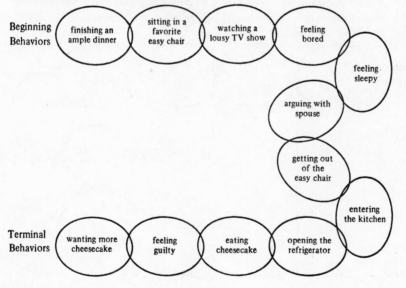

ALTERNATE ACTIVITY SHEET

SUBSTITUTE ACTIVITIES

Pleasant Activities   1. _____

2. _____

3. _____

Necessary Activities   1. _____

2. _____

3. _____

Situations when used   1. _____

2. _____

3. _____

4. _____

5. _____

6. _____

7. _____

BEHAVIOR CHAIN

Identify the links in your eating response chain on the following diagram. Draw a line through the chain where it was interrupted. Add the link you substituted and the new chain of behaviors this substitution started.

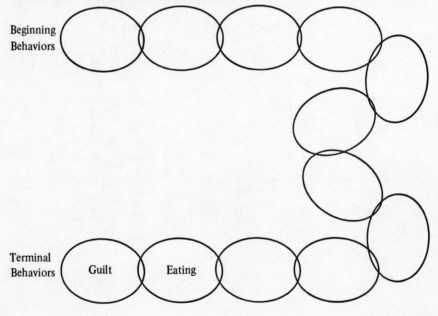

Beginning
Behaviors

Terminal
Behaviors   Guilt   Eating

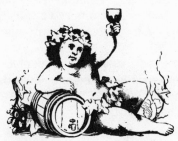

Lesson Five

Behavioral Analysis, Progress, and Problem Solving

WEIGH-IN AND HOMEWORK.

Weigh yourself and record your weight on your Master Data Sheet. Graph your weight change for the past week.

Compare your weight loss with the average weight loss line of one pound per week.

Check your homework.

—Is your Lesson Four Food Diary complete? Yes_____ No_____

—Did you fill in the Eating Ratio column each day? Yes_____ No_____

—Is your Eating Place record completed? Yes_____
No_____

—Did you define a behavior chain and fill out your Alternate
Activity Sheet? Yes_____ No_____

—Did you keep a record of situations where you were able to
break a behavior chain? Yes_____ No_____

Give yourself credit towards your refund on your Homework Credit
Sheet.

REVIEW.

The Food Diary will continue to be one of your most valuable tools for
some time. This is because it gives immediate feedback about all of your
eating behaviors. The sooner after a meal you fill it out, the more effective
it will be in sensitizing you to your style of eating and the content of
your meals.

We have introduced many specific techniques to change the act
of eating. Two of them you were asked to use this past week were keeping
the Eating Place Record, and trying the eating delay technique of putting
your utensils down after each bite.

Consider How You Are Doing.

• Are you still keeping track? Yes_____ No_____

• Do you remember why you are doing these exercises?
Yes_____ No_____

• Are you continuing to do the cue elimination exercises:

	Yes	No
1. Eating in your Designated Appropriate Eating Place?	_____	_____
2. Sitting at a different place at the table?	_____	_____
3. When eating, *only* eating?	_____	_____
4. Reducing visual cues—food stored out of sight, in opaque containers, etc.?	_____	_____
5. Alternate foods?	_____	_____
6. All serving dishes off the table?	_____	_____

If not, refer back to Lesson Two, review the techniques, and try again.

If you feel these are established habits, you can stop recording
them on the feedback forms. If you want additional feedback during the
five-week Maintenance period, make an extra copy of the forms.

New behaviors are fragile and must be practiced over and over until they become habits. As we emphasized in the first lessons, weight loss without maintenance is worthless. The object of these exercises is to introduce new eating behaviors to you and have you *over*-practice until they become habits. Later in this lesson we will introduce a technique to help you keep track of your new eating behaviors and give you direct feedback on your progress and maintenance during the next five weeks.

Behavior Chains and Alternate Activities.   In Lesson Four the concept was introduced that behaviors are linked together in chains; that is, one behavior can make the immediately following behavior more or less probable. For example, buying a bag of potato chips increases the probability of a snack. In this case a behavior prior to the snack influences the probability of the snack.

We developed this conceptual framework and demonstrated how it can be used to control food intake. The concept is quite simple. A behavior such as eating has an immediately antecedent behavior such as opening the refrigerator. This behavior, too, has an antecedent, entering the kitchen, and so forth, back to finishing dinner an hour before and feeling full. If the chain of behaviors is broken at any point, it will probably not continue to the final behavior in the chain—eating. The earlier the break in the chain, the easier it is to unlink the chain of activities. The interventions (breaks) can be quite simple. In the example given in last lesson, we substituted an exciting book for a dull T-V show, a nap for boredom, and an alternate food for cheesecake.

Many times the behavior chain cannot be identified, or you will find yourself on the brink of the terminal behavior of eating before you are even aware of heading toward food. In this case we proposed directly substituting an activity for eating. These activities were of two types: things that you have to do, such as errands, washing dishes, and paying bills; and things that are enjoyable, such as hobbies, sleep, sex, taking a walk, and music. We suggested you begin a substitute activity as soon as you have a craving for food. Another strategy was simply to interpose time between you and a snack. Set a clock or cooking timer to help you interject progressively longer periods of time between the links in the behavior chain.

The assignment last week had three parts:

1. You were to write down a behavior chain, starting with eating (the terminal end behavior) and working backwards to the beginning. You were asked to look for a weak link in the chain where you could substitute an alternate activity. The earlier in the chain you make this substitution, the easier it will be to break the chain.

2. You were to write down at least three necessary and three pleasant activities that could be substituted for eating in a behavioral chain.

3. Finally, you were to substitute an activity from your list for a link in the chain, or for an inappropriate eating episode or snack.

Have You Been Able to Assimilate This?

- The theory of behavior chains? (Page 65)
- Alternate activities, their definition or use? (Page 67)
- Why or how to substitute alternate activities for antecedent events to disrupt behavior chains? (Page 68)
- What were some of the occasions where you made a successful substitution?

    1. _____

    2. _____

- Were there some additional substitutions you could have made?

    1. _____

    2. _____

These techniques can be very useful if they are systematically applied to your inappropriate eating. Many of us are trapped into daily habit patterns that lead to eating—to consumption of food that we would not even be tempted by if it weren't for the circumstances that lead up to it. This technique of changing behavior patterns is the way to liberate yourself from that unnecessary eating.

NEW TECHNIQUE: PROBLEM SOLVING, OR BECOMING YOUR OWN THERAPIST.

The problems we have worked on up to now are universal; everyone with a weight problem has them. The solutions we have suggested are useful for everyone.

This week we want you to learn how to identify and solve your particular problems: to become your own behavior therapist. When you have finished this program, you will have the ability to spot an eating problem and solve it. Everyone has some problem eating behaviors which are unique, and some new ones will develop in the future—it is inevitable. However, if you apply the techniques taught here, you will have the skills to solve any eating problem.

Behavior modification programs are only an organized way of very specifically defining and solving problems. For example, we have defined the problem of eating too rapidly and have offered two solutions: introducing a delay by putting down your fork after each bite; and adding a two-minute delay between courses during the meal. Breaking down the problem-solving process into separate steps is useful, both from the standpoint of figuring out what to do with the problems and also to help reanalyze the problems when a solution does not work.

The steps in solving behavioral problems are easily separated into five categories:

1. ***Observation and Long-term Goal Definition.*** This means looking at the big problem to try to see what can be arranged. An example is using a Food Diary to look at eating behaviors, with an over-all goal of losing weight.

2. ***Identification and Definition of Specific Well-Defined Small Problems, or Short-termed Goal Setting.*** These problems are the small steps you take toward a long-term goal. Each step is to be taken in connection with the behaviors you have identified during your observations; for example, identifying the problem of eating too large a breakfast every day when you look at your Food Diary.

3. ***Creative Problem Solving, or Brainstorming.*** This is a method of uncritically producing solutions to the defined problem. There are usually many ways to solve behavioral problems. No way is right or wrong; some ways are more direct, some faster, but many will be effective. For example, several techniques might be used to modify that large daily breakfast. We might propose:

   a. Slow down, introduce a two-minute delay after the toast and coffee;

   b. Eliminate cues—for example, by only eating at the breakfast table (not at the open refrigerator), and not reading the paper at breakfast;

   c. Substitute lower-calorie foods—for example, artificial sweeteners, thinner bread, and non-fat milk;

   d. Elimination techniques—for example, eliminating a food like bacon, or slowly decreasing the portion size of a food like bread.

An almost endless list can be made for any specific problem. Most of the time several techniques may be used at once.

4. **Decision Making.** At this point, you choose the plan or plans that seem to be most appropriate. In general, try to change behaviors only a few steps at a time. It is important not to go too fast or to change too many things at one time; you'll fail and become discouraged when things don't change. You should plan to succeed at least 80 percent of the time.

5. **Feedback and Evaluation.** This is one of the most important steps. If you do not periodically evaluate your progress, you will not know when you are successful. If you find your plan is not working, don't charge yourself with lack of will power or a moral defect; more likely, you didn't choose a good plan, or it is too big a change for one step, or you have not identified the problem. Look over the whole problem-solving process again, and don't be afraid to change plans if something isn't working. Be creative in your approach.

As part of the assignment for today, you will transfer the information from your Week One and Week Four Food Diaries to a Behavioral Analysis Form. This side-by-side display of your beginning and modified eating patterns will show you how much your eating behaviors have changed during the first three weeks of the program.

The fastest way to accomplish this is to ask someone to help you by reading off the columns of items from your Food Diaries. For example (using the Week One Sample Food Diary), under "time," they will read off "6:45, 7:13, 9:45, etc." On the Behavioral Analysis Form, mark the appropriate squares on the chart labeled "Time of Eating." When you have put all of the times on the chart, go on to the "Minutes Spent Eating," "Hunger," "Body Position," etc. When you have completed your Week One Food Diary, go on to your Week Four Food Diary. You will probably be surprised to see how many basic habits you have changed in three weeks.

Look over your Food Diaries and Behavioral Analysis Forms and define a specific small problem. Ask the person who helped you with the Analysis Form to help you look for problems. Make a list of all of the possible solutions that come to mind for *one* specific problem. Make sure you include some method of self-evaluation or feedback with the solution so you can monitor your progress. This can be a graph, a table, gold stars, or anything that will keep track of the behavior you are trying to change. If you have no way of measuring your problem behavior, you will never know if you are successful.

Among the materials for this week is a blank Behavioral Prescription Sheet and a sample sheet filled out for a hypothetical problem. Fill out your sheet with the problem and solutions you decide on today. Ask a friend or family member to read it over and help you with solutions to your newly defined eating problem, and ask them to witness it by signing on the line labeled "Consultant."

The goal of this exercise is to gain experience and expertise in defining problems and in planning solutions. Make a commitment today to work on a definite problem for the coming five weeks, in addition to continuing to practice the new behaviors you have developed in the first five weeks of the program. In Lesson Six, the first lesson after the Maintenance period, you will review your problems, solutions, and successes. If, during the Maintenance period, you find you have eliminated the problem you define today, define and work on another one. The more the better.

Remember to keep the defined problem very specific. If the problem is one that has already been discussed, for example, eating in one place, and you want to continue working on it for the next weeks, that is fine. Your observations, defined problems, alternative solutions, ultimate plan, and method of feedback evaluation should all be very clearly spelled out on the Behavioral Prescription Sheet.

MAINTENANCE.

The final form to begin filling out today is a Daily Behavior Checklist, which will help you keep track of your new behaviors. Read it over each morning before breakfast to remind yourself of the specific techniques we have discussed. In the evening after dinner, rate yourself on a scale of 1–3 on how well you carried out each of the techniques during the day. This is a subjective measurement on your part; there are no right or wrong answers. But consistency in your self-evaluation is important if it is to be meaningful.

The five-week Maintenance period begins this week. During the coming five weeks practice what you have learned in the first five lessons. Carefully weigh yourself each week at the same time of the day and keep your Master Data Sheet and graph up to date. This feedback about your progress is vital to maintaining your program.

The five-week practice period is a time for you to consolidate your learning before you go on to more techniques. Although it is tempting, *DO NOT* jump ahead to Lesson Six—it would only be asking for failure. You have a whole lifetime to lose weight, and it is important to go about it at a speed that virtually guarantees success. This five-week period will also give you a preview of how hard it will be to continue your new eating skills when there is not the pressure and incentive of a new lesson and new techniques to learn each week.

When you read Lesson Six (in five weeks), you will go over your Maintenance Food Diaries and Daily Behavior Checklists, and you will assess how well you were able to maintain your behavior changes. During this five-week period you should try to master all of the concepts presented in the first five weeks of the program. Use it to practice what you have learned.

HOMEWORK.

A. Transfer the information from your Lesson One and Lesson Four Food Diaries to your Behavioral Analysis form. Compare the patterns for these two weeks.

B. Food Diaries for Lesson Five.

C. Daily Behavior Checklist for Lesson Five.

D. Food Diaries for Maintenance, Weeks 1–5.

E. Daily Behavior Checklist for Maintenance weeks 1–5.

F. Problem solving. Solve at least the problem defined on the Behavioral Prescription Sheet today. Use the blank columns of the Food Diary for individual problems you define during the five-week Maintenance period.

G. Master Data Sheet. Plot your weekly weight change for the next five weeks. If necessary, arrange an individual time each week to be weighed.

H. Maintenance: PRACTICE, PRACTICE, PRACTICE!

FOOD DIARY – Lesson Five

Day of Week _____   Name_____

Time	M/S	H	Food Type and Quantity	Eating Ratio
6:00				
11:00				
4:00				
9:00				

FOOD DIARY – Lesson Five

Day of Week _____   Name_____

Time	M/S	H	Food Type and Quantity	Eating Ratio
6:00				
11:00				
4:00				
9:00				

FOOD DIARY – Lesson Five

Day of Week _____   Name_____

Time	M/S	H	Food Type and Quantity	Eating Ratio
6:00				
11:00				
4:00				
9:00				

FOOD DIARY – Lesson Five

Day of Week _____   Name_____

Time	M/S	H	Food Type and Quantity	Eating Ratio
6:00				
11:00				
4:00				
9:00				

FOOD DIARY – Lesson Five

Day of Week _____   Name_____

Time	M/S	H	Food Type and Quantity	Eating Ratio
6:00				
11:00				
4:00				
9:00				

FOOD DIARY – Lesson Five

Day of Week _____   Name_____

Time	M/S	H	Food Type and Quantity	Eating Ratio
6:00				
11:00				
4:00				
9:00				

FOOD DIARY – Lesson Five

Day of Week _____   Name_____

Time	M/S	H	Food Type and Quantity	Eating Ratio
6:00				
11:00				
4:00				
9:00				

DAILY BEHAVIOR CHECKLIST – Lesson Five,

Points: Most of the time, or yes = 3
          Sometimes   = 2
          Not at all, or no   = 1

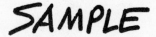

Days of the Week

	1	2	3	4	5	6	7
1. Daily Checklist							
a. Morning review (3 if I read the checklist)	3	3	3	3	3	3	3
b. Evening scoring (3 if I rated myself)	3	3	3	3	3	3	3
2. Food Diary							
a. Recording my food	2	3	3	3	3	3	2
3. Cue Elimination							
a. Designated eating place	2	3	2	3	3	3	1
b. Change place at table	2	3	3	3	3	3	3
c. Only eating when eating	2	3	2	3	3	3	2
d. Reduce visual cues-storage, opaque containers	2	2	2	3	3	3	3
e. Serving dishes off the table	2	3	3	3	3	2	3
f. Junk food out of sight	2	2	3	3	3	3	3
4. Eating Delay							
a. Utensils down between mouthfuls	1	2	3	3	3	3	3
b. Swallowing each forkful before adding the next	2	2	2	2	2	3	3
c. Chewing slowly and thoroughly	2	2	3	3	3	3	3
d. Enjoying the meal	2	2	3	3	3	3	3
e. Programming a delay in the meal	2	2	2	2	2	3	3
5. Becoming My Own Therapist							
a. Individual problem solving	3	3	3	3	3	3	3
DAILY TOTALS	32	38	40	43	43	44	41

Total Points For the Week ___281___   Weight ___190___

DAILY BEHAVIOR CHECKLIST – Lesson Five,

Points: Most of the time, or yes = 3
         Sometimes   = 2
         Not at all, or no   = 1

Days of the Week

	1	2	3	4	5	6	7
1. *Daily Checklist* a. Morning review (3 if I read the checklist)							
b. Evening scoring (3 if I rated myself)							
2. *Food Diary* a. Recording my food							
3. *Cue Elimination* a. Designated eating place							
b. Change place at table							
c. Only eating when eating							
d. Reduce visual cues-storage, opaque containers							
e. Serving dishes off the table							
f. Junk food out of sight							
4. *Eating Delay* a. Utensils down between mouthfuls							
b. Swallowing each forkful before adding the next							
c. Chewing slowly and thoroughly							
d. Enjoying the meal							
e. Programming a delay in the meal							
5. *Becoming My Own Therapist* a. Individual problem solving							
DAILY TOTALS							

Total Points For the Week _____   Weight _____

BEHAVIORAL PRESCRIPTION SHEET — SAMPLE

Name _____ FRED SCHWARTZ _____

Partner _____ MARY SMITH _____

Problem _____ POOR EATIN HABIT OF SNACKING EVERY
HOUR FROM 3:00 PM TO 12:00 MIDNIGHT _____

Solutions ① TAKE SNACK TO DESIGNATED AREA.
② REMOVE SNACK FOODS FROM THE HOUSE.
③ EAT TWO CARROTS BEFORE EVERY SNACK.
④ SNACK ONLY AT ODD NUMBERED HOURS
FROM 11:00 A.M. TO 11:00 P.M.
⑤ DO TWENTY SITUPS BEFORE EACH SNACK.

Plan ① START CUTTING DOWN BY SNACKING EVERY OTHER
HOUR.
② EACH OF THESE SNACKS WILL BE PRECEDED BY
TWO CARROTS.

Feedback _____ GRAPH OF SNACKS PER DAY FOR TWO WEEKS. _____

Consultation _____ MARY SMITH _____

BEHAVIORAL PRESCRIPTION SHEET —

Name _____

Partner _____

Problem _____
_____
_____
_____

Solutions_____
_____
_____
_____
_____
_____
_____
_____
_____

Plan _____
_____
_____
_____
_____
_____

Feedback_____
_____
_____

Consultation _____

SAMPLE

BEHAVIORAL ANALYSIS FORM

TIME OF EATING

Indicate the time of day for each eating episode during the week by making a mark in the square above the appropriate time of day. Start with the bottom row of boxes. If you have a second eating episode during the week within that time range, indicate it by filling in the next box in that column. For example, if you had a snack at 10:30 am, you would fill in the first box in the time of day column labeled "10-11 am." If the next day, you had breakfast at 10:15 am, you would blacken in the next box up in that same column. If that same day, you had a snack at 10:50 am, you would indicate this by marking the third box in the same column. When you have entered an entire week's eating pattern in these boxes, you will have a graph which shows the distribution of your eating during the week.

Lesson One / Lesson Four — Eating Episodes grids (Time of Day, AM / PM / AM)

MINUTES SPENT EATING

Indicate the duration of *each* of your eating episodes by making a tally mark on the line under the appropriate heading — "meal" or "snack". For example, if breakfast took seven minutes, put a mark under the word "meal" on the line labeled "5-10 minutes." If you had a mid-afternoon snack that lasted 13 minutes, put a mark under "snack" on the line labeled "10-15 minutes." If you had six meals, each 5-10 minutes long, you would have six talleys (卌 I) in the meal column on the line marked 5-10 minutes.

Lesson One

	Meal	Snack
0-5 minutes.	卌 I	卌 卌 II
5-10 minutes.	IIII	卌 IIII
10-15 minutes.	卌 I	II
15-20 minutes.	III	
20-30 minutes.	I	
over 30 minutes.		

Lesson Four

	Meal	Snack
0-5 minutes.		II
5-10 minutes.	I	IIII
10-15 minutes.		
15-20 minutes.	卌 I	
20-30 minutes.	卌 IIII	
over 30 minutes.	卌	

(Adapted from and used by permission of Leonard S. Levitz, Ph.D., and Henry A. Jordan, M.D., University of Pennsylvania School of Medicine, "Analysis of Food Intake and Energy Expenditure," Copyright, 1973.)

BEHAVIORAL ANALYSIS FORM

TIME OF EATING

Indicate the time of day for each eating episode during the week by making a mark in the square above the appropriate time of day. Start with the bottom row of boxes. If you have a second eating episode during the week within that time range, indicate it by filling in the next box in that column. For example, if you had a snack at 10:30 am, you would fill in the first box in the time of day column labeled "10-11 am." If the next day, you had breakfast at 10:15 am, you would blacken in the next box up in that same column. If that same day, you had a snack at 10:50 am, you would indicate this by marking the third box in the same column. When you have entered an entire week's eating pattern in these boxes, you will have a graph which shows the distribution of your eating during the week.

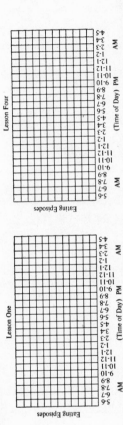

MINUTES SPENT EATING

Lesson One

	Meal	Snack
0-5 minutes.......	_____	_____
5-10 minutes.......	_____	_____
10-15 minutes......	_____	_____
15-20 minutes......	_____	_____
20-30 minutes......	_____	_____
over 30 minutes.....	_____	_____

Lesson Four

	Meal	Snack
0-5 minutes.......	_____	_____
5-10 minutes......	_____	_____
10-15 minutes.....	_____	_____
15-20 minutes.....	_____	_____
20-30 minutes.....	_____	_____
over 30 minutes....	_____	_____

Indicate the duration of *each* of your eating episodes by making a tally mark on the line under the appropriate heading — "meal" or "snack" For example, if breakfast took seven minutes, put a mark under the word "meal" on the line labeled "5-10 minutes." If you had a midafternoon snack that lasted 13 minutes, put a mark under "snack" on the line labeled "10-15 minutes." If you had six meals, each 5-10 minutes long, you would have six tallies (卌 I) in the meal column on the line marked 5-10 minutes.

(Adapted from and used by permission of Leonard S. Levitz, Ph.D., and Henry A. Jordon, M.D., University of Pennsylvania School of Medicine, "Analysis of Food Intake and Energy Expenditure," Copyright, 1973.)

BEHAVIORAL ANALYSIS FORM
DEGREE OF HUNGER

SAMPLE

	Lesson One		Lesson Four	
	Meal	Snack	Meal	Snack
0 – none	THI I	THI THI III	II	II
1 – some	THI IIII	THI II	THI THI	IIII
2 – hungry	THI	II	THI II	
3 – extreme			II	

Put a tally mark on the appropriate line to indicate the degree of hunger you felt at the beginning of every episode of eating during the week. For example, if you had a snack and were not hungry, put a mark under snack on the line labeled "none." If you felt like you were starving to death when you had dinner, put a mark under "meal" on the line labeled "extreme." (Note: Use the same numbers that appear on your Week One Food Diary.)

BODY POSITION WHILE EATING

	Lesson One			Lesson Four	
	Meal	Snack		Meal	Snack
Walking	IIII	THI II	Walking		I
Standing	THI	THI III	Standing	I	I
Sitting	THI THI I	IIII	Sitting	THI THI THI THI	IIII
Lying Down	I	III	Lying Down		

Put a tally mark on the appropriate line to indicate your body position during each episode of eating for the week. For example, if you had a snack while walking around the grocery store, put a mark under "snack" on the line labeled "walking". If you ate dinner lying in bed watching television, put a mark under "meal" on the line labeled "lying down."

ACTIVITIES WHILE EATING

	Lesson One		Lesson Four	
	Meal	Snack	Meal	Snack
None: only eating	I	II	III	
Talking		IIII	THI THI III	III
Listening to music or radio		II	IIII	
Reading a book or paper	THI II	III		
Watching television	THI I	THI II		I
Cooking-working in kitchen				
Working-studying	THI I	IIII	I	II
Other				

Put a tally mark on the appropriate line to indicate activities that are associated with your episodes of eating. For example, if you ate lunch while working at your desk, put a mark under "meal" on the line labeled "working." If you had a snack while preparing dinner, put a mark under the "snack" column on the line labeled "cooking."

(Adapted from and used by permission of Leonard S. Levitz, Ph.D., and Henry A. Jordan, M.D., University of Pennsylvania School of Medicine, "Analysis of Food Intake and Energy Expenditure," Copyright, 1973.)

BEHAVIORAL ANALYSIS FORM

DEGREE OF HUNGER

	Lesson One			Lesson Four	
	Meal	Snack		Meal	Snack
0 – none	_____	_____	...0 – none	_____	_____
1 – some	_____	_____	...1 – some	_____	_____
2 – hungry...	_____	_____	...2 – hungry ...	_____	_____
3 – extreme...	_____	_____	... 3 – extreme ...	_____	_____

Put a tally mark on the appropriate line to indicate the degree of hunger you felt at the beginning of every episode of eating during the week. For example, if you had a snack and were not hungry, put a mark under snack on the line labeled "none." If you felt like you were starving to death when you had dinner, put a mark under "meal" on the line labeled "extreme." (Note: Use the same numbers that appear on your Week One Food Diary.)

BODY POSITION WHILE EATING

	Lesson One				Lesson Four	
	Meal	Snack			Meal	Snack
Walking	_____	_____		Walking	_____	_____
Standing ...	_____	_____		Standing ...	_____	_____
Sitting	_____	_____		Sitting	_____	_____
Lying Down.	_____	_____		Lying Down.	_____	_____

Put a tally mark on the appropriate line to indicate your body position during each episode of eating for the week. For example, if you had a snack while walking around the grocery store, put a mark under "snack" on the line labeled "walking". If you ate dinner lying in bed watching television, put a mark under "meal" on the line labeled "lying down."

ACTIVITIES WHILE EATING

	Lesson One		Lesson Four	
	Meal	Snack	Meal	Snack
None: only eating	_____	_____	_____	_____
Talking.................	_____	_____	_____	_____
Listening to music or radio.....	_____	_____	_____	_____
Reading a book or paper......	_____	_____	_____	_____
Watching television..........	_____	_____	_____	_____
Cooking-working in kitchen....	_____	_____	_____	_____
Working-studying...........	_____	_____	_____	_____
Other	_____	_____	_____	_____

Put a tally mark on the appropriate line to indicate activities that are associated with your episodes of eating. For example, if you ate lunch while working at your desk, put a mark under "meal" on the line labeled "working." If you had a snack while preparing dinner, put a mark under the "snack" column on the line labeled "cooking."

FOOD DIARY — **Maintenance Week One**

Day of Week _____   Name_____

Time	M/S	H	Food Type and Quantity	Eating Ratio
6:00				
11:00				
4:00				
9:00				

FOOD DIARY – Maintenance Week One

Day of Week _____   Name_____

Time	M/S	H	Food Type and Quantity	Eating Ratio
6:00				
11:00				
4:00				
9:00				

FOOD DIARY – **Maintenance Week One**

Day of Week _____   Name_____

Time	M/S	H	Food Type and Quantity	Eating Ratio
6:00				
11:00				
4:00				
9:00				

FOOD DIARY – Maintenance Week One

Day of Week _____   Name_____

Time	M/S	H	Food Type and Quantity	Eating Ratio
6:00				
11:00				
4:00				
9:00				

FOOD DIARY – Maintenance Week One

Day of Week _____   Name_____

Time	M/S	H	Food Type and Quantity	Eating Ratio
6:00				
11:00				
4:00				
9:00				

FOOD DIARY – Maintenance Week One

Day of Week _____   Name_____

Time	M/S	H	Food Type and Quantity	Eating Ratio
6:00				
11:00				
4:00				
9:00				

FOOD DIARY – Maintenance Week One

Day of Week _____   Name_____

Time	M/S	H	Food Type and Quantity	Eating Ratio
6:00				
11:00				
4:00				
9:00				

DAILY BEHAVIOR CHECKLIST – Maintenance Week One

Points: Most of the time, or yes = 3
Sometimes   = 2
Not at all, or no   = 1

Days of the Week

	1	2	3	4	5	6	7
1. *Daily Checklist* a. Morning review (3 if I read the checklist)							
b. Evening scoring (3 if I rated myself)							
2. *Food Diary* a. Recording my food							
3. *Cue Elimination* a. Designated eating place							
b. Change place at table							
c. Only eating when eating							
d. Reduce visual cues-storage, opaque containers							
e. Serving dishes off the table							
f. Junk food out of sight							
4. *Eating Delay* a. Utensils down between mouthfuls							
b. Swallowing each forkful before adding the next							
c. Chewing slowly and thoroughly							
d. Enjoying the meal							
e. Programming a delay in the meal							
5. *Becoming My Own Therapist* a. Individual problem solving							
DAILY TOTALS							

Total Points For the Week _____   Weight _____

FOOD DIARY – Maintenance Week Two

Day of Week _____   Name_____

Time	M/S	H	Food Type and Quantity	Eating Ratio
6:00				
11:00				
4:00				
9:00				

FOOD DIARY -- Maintenance Week Two

Day of Week _____   Name_____

Time	M/S	H	Food Type and Quantity	Eating Ratio
6:00				
11:00				
4:00				
9:00				

FOOD DIARY – Maintenance Week Two

Day of Week _____   Name_____

Time	M/S	H	Food Type and Quantity	Eating Ratio
6:00				
11:00				
4:00				
9:00				

FOOD DIARY – Maintenance Week Two

Day of Week _____   Name_____

Time	M/S	H	Food Type and Quantity	Eating Ratio
6:00				
11:00				
4:00				
9:00				

FOOD DIARY – Maintenance Week Two

Day of Week _____   Name_____

Time	M/S	H	Food Type and Quantity	Eating Ratio
6:00				
11:00				
4:00				
9:00				

FOOD DIARY – Maintenance Week Two

Day of Week _____   Name_____

Time	M/S	H	Food Type and Quantity	Eating Ratio
6:00				
11:00				
4:00				
9:00				

FOOD DIARY – Maintenance Week Two

Day of Week _____   Name_____

Time	M/S	H	Food Type and Quantity	Eating Ratio
6:00				
11:00				
4:00				
9:00				

DAILY BEHAVIOR CHECKLIST – Maintenance Week Two

Points: Most of the time, or yes = 3
Sometimes = 2
Not at all, or no = 1

Days of the Week

	1	2	3	4	5	6	7
1. *Daily Checklist* a. Morning review (3 if I read the checklist)							
b. Evening scoring (3 if I rated myself)							
2. *Food Diary* a. Recording my food							
3. *Cue Elimination* a. Designated eating place							
b. Change place at table							
c. Only eating when eating							
d. Reduce visual cues-storage, opaque containers							
e. Serving dishes off the table							
f. Junk food out of sight							
4. *Eating Delay* a. Utensils down between mouthfuls							
b. Swallowing each forkful before adding the next							
c. Chewing slowly and thoroughly							
d. Enjoying the meal							
e. Programming a delay in the meal							
5. *Becoming My Own Therapist* a. Individual problem solving							
DAILY TOTALS							

Total Points For the Week ⎯⎯⎯⎯⎯⎯   Weight ⎯⎯⎯⎯⎯

FOOD DIARY – Maintenance Week Three

Day of Week _____   Name_____

Time	M/S	H	Food Type and Quantity	Eating Ratio
6:00				
11:00				
4:00				
9:00				

FOOD DIARY — Maintenance Week Three

Day of Week _____   Name_____

Time	M/S	H	Food Type and Quantity	Eating Ratio
6:00				
11:00				
4:00				
9:00				

FOOD DIARY – Maintenance Week Three

Day of Week _____   Name_____

Time	M/S	H	Food Type and Quantity	Eating Ratio
6:00				
11:00				
4:00				
9:00				

FOOD DIARY – Maintenance Week Three

Day of Week _____   Name_____

Time	M/S	H	Food Type and Quantity	Eating Ratio
6:00				
11:00				
4:00				
9:00				

FOOD DIARY – Maintenance Week Three

Day of Week _____   Name_____

Time	M/S	H	Food Type and Quantity	Eating Ratio
6:00				
11:00				
4:00				
9:00				

FOOD DIARY – Maintenance Week Three

Day of Week _____   Name_____

Time	M/S	H	Food Type and Quantity	Eating Ratio
6:00				
11:00				
4:00				
9:00				

FOOD DIARY – Maintenance Week Three

Day of Week _____   Name_____

Time	M/S	H	Food Type and Quantity	Eating Ratio
6:00				
11:00				
4:00				
9:00				

DAILY BEHAVIOR CHECKLIST — Maintenance Week Three

Points: Most of the time, or yes = 3
          Sometimes   = 2
          Not at all, or no   = 1

Days of the Week

	1	2	3	4	5	6	7
1. *Daily Checklist* a. Morning review (3 if I read the checklist)							
b. Evening scoring (3 if I rated myself)							
2. *Food Diary* a. Recording my food							
3. *Cue Elimination* a. Designated eating place							
b. Change place at table							
c. Only eating when eating							
d. Reduce visual cues-storage, opaque containers							
e. Serving dishes off the table							
f. Junk food out of sight							

4. *Eating Delay*
  a. Utensils down between
   mouthfuls							

b. Swallowing each forkful before adding the next							
c. Chewing slowly and thoroughly							
d. Enjoying the meal							
e. Programming a delay in the meal							
5. *Becoming My Own Therapist* a. Individual problem solving							
DAILY TOTALS							

Total Points For the Week ———————   Weight ————————

FOOD DIARY – Maintenance Week Four

Day of Week _____   Name_____

Time	M/S	H	Food Type and Quantity	Eating Ratio
6:00				
11:00				
4:00				
9:00				

FOOD DIARY – **Maintenance Week Four**

Day of Week _____   Name_____

Time	M/S	H	Food Type and Quantity	Eating Ratio
6:00				
11:00				
4:00				
9:00				

FOOD DIARY – Maintenance Week Four

Day of Week _____   Name_____

Time	M/S	H	Food Type and Quantity	Eating Ratio
6:00				
11:00				
4:00				
9:00				

FOOD DIARY – **Maintenance Week Four**

Day of Week _____   Name_____

Time	M/S	H	Food Type and Quantity	Eating Ratio
6:00				
11:00				
4:00				
9:00				

FOOD DIARY — Maintenance Week Four

Day of Week:_____   Name_____

Time	M/S	H	Food Type and Quantity	Eating Ratio
6:00				
11:00				
4:00				
9:00				

FOOD DIARY – Maintenance Week Four

Day of Week _____   Name_____

Time	M/S	H	Food Type and Quantity	Eating Ratio
6:00				
11:00				
4:00				
9:00				

FOOD DIARY – Maintenance Week Four

Day of Week _____   Name_____

Time	M/S	H	Food Type and Quantity	Eating Ratio
6:00				
11:00				
4:00				
9:00				

DAILY BEHAVIOR CHECKLIST – Maintenance Week Four

Points: Most of the time, or yes = 3
Sometimes   = 2
Not at all, or no   = 1

Days of the Week

	1	2	3	4	5	6	7
1. *Daily Checklist* a. Morning review (3 if I read the checklist)							
b. Evening scoring (3 if I rated myself)							
2. *Food Diary* a. Recording my food							
3. *Cue Elimination* a. Designated eating place							
b. Change place at table							
c. Only eating when eating							
d. Reduce visual cues-storage, opaque containers							
e. Serving dishes off the table							
f. Junk food out of sight							

4. *Eating Delay*
  a. Utensils down between
    mouthfuls							

b. Swallowing each forkful before adding the next							
c. Chewing slowly and thoroughly							
d. Enjoying the meal							
e. Programming a delay in the meal							
5. *Becoming My Own Therapist* a. Individual problem solving							
DAILY TOTALS							

Total Points For the Week ＿＿＿＿＿＿   Weight ＿＿＿＿＿

This is the final week of your Maintenance program. This practice period of five weeks was included in the behavior change program for a specific reason: new behaviors tend to fade away and are forgotten if they are not practiced. During the past month, you have kept a Food Diary and a Behavior Checklist. Monitoring your eating behaviors daily to give yourself feedback, and to tell yourself how well you are practicing your new eating habits is essential while you are developing new habits.

For this final Maintenance Week, keep a complete Food Diary. It is similar to the one you filled out during the fourth lesson. You will go over it in detail next lesson with a Behavioral Analysis Form and determine how well you have maintained your new eating skills—and how close they are to becoming habits.

FOOD DIARY – Maintenance Week Five

Day of Week_____   Name_____

Time	Min Spent Eating	M/S	H	Body Position	Activity While Eating	Location of Eating	Food Type and Quantity	Ratio
6:00								
11:00								
4:00								
9:00								

FOOD DIARY – Maintenance Week Five

Day of Week_____   Name_____

Time	Min Spent Eating	M/S	H	Body Position	Activity While Eating	Location of Eating	Food Type and Quantity	Ratio
6:00								
11:00								
4:00								
9:00								

FOOD DIARY – Maintenance Week Five

Day of Week_____   Name_____

Time	Min Spent Eating	M/S	H	Body Position	Activity While Eating	Location of Eating	Food Type and Quantity	Ratio
6:00								
11:00								
4:00								
9:00								

FOOD DIARY – **Maintenance Week Five**

Day of Week_____   Name_____

Time	Min Spent Eating	M/S	H	Body Position	Activity While Eating	Location of Eating	Food Type and Quantity	Ratio
6:00								
11:00								
4:00								
9:00								

FOOD DIARY – **Maintenance Week Five**

Day of Week_____   Name_____

Time	Min Spent Eating	M/S	H	Body Position	Activity While Eating	Location of Eating	Food Type and Quantity	Ratio
6:00								
11:00								
4:00								
9:00								

FOOD DIARY – Maintenance Week Five

Day of Week_____   Name_____

Time	Min Spent Eating	M/S	H	Body Position	Activity While Eating	Location of Eating	Food Type and Quantity	Ratio
6:00								
11:00								
4:00								
9:00								

FOOD DIARY – Maintenance Week Five

Day of Week_____   Name_____

Time	Min Spent Eating	M/S	H	Body Position	Activity While Eating	Location of Eating	Food Type and Quantity	Ratio
6:00								
11:00								
4:00								
9:00								

DAILY BEHAVIOR CHECKLIST — Maintenance Week Five

Points: Most of the time, or yes = 3
          Sometimes   = 2
          Not at all, or no   = 1

Days of the Week

	1	2	3	4	5	6	7
1. *Daily Checklist* a. Morning review (3 if I read the checklist)							
b. Evening scoring (3 if I rated myself)							
2. *Food Diary* a. Recording my food							
3. *Cue Elimination* a. Designated eating place							
b. Change place at table							
c. Only eating when eating							
d. Reduce visual cues-storage, opaque containers							
e. Serving dishes off the table							
f. Junk food out of sight							
4. *Eating Delay* a. Utensils down between mouthfuls							
b. Swallowing each forkful before adding the next							
c. Chewing slowly and thoroughly							
d. Enjoying the meal							
e. Programming a delay in the meal							
5. *Becoming My Own Therapist* a. Individual problem solving							
DAILY TOTALS							

Total Points For the Week _____   Weight _____

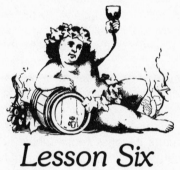

Lesson Six

Pre-Planning

WEIGH-IN AND HOMEWORK.

Weigh yourself and record your weight on your Master Data Sheet. Graph your weight change and compare it with the "average" line on your Master Data Sheet.

     Check your homework, and record it on your Homework Credit Schedule.

     —Is your Maintenance Week Five Food Diary complete? Yes_____ No_____

     —Have you completed your Behavioral Prescription Sheet from Week Five? Yes_____ No_____

     —Did you fill in the Daily Behavior Checklist for Maintenance Week Five? Yes_____ No_____

MAINTENANCE.

Today you are starting the second half of the ten weeks of instruction in the *Learning to Eat* program. A large number of impulse-eating control methods were presented during the first five weeks of instruction. The five-week period just concluded was for Maintenance, or practice. It was as important as the learning periods. Without the practice period, people become overloaded with new techniques, and soon stop doing some of those introduced earlier to make time for the more recently introduced ones. If you did not learn how to follow a Maintenance program, you would end up with nothing to show for your efforts.

You started to keep a Daily Behavior Checklist at the end of Lesson Five. This served as a *subjective* measure of Maintenance. Each morning you were to read it over before breakfast to remind yourself of the behaviors stressed in the course. In the evening, after dinner, you were to rate yourself on your progress in developing the new behaviors. Although it may seem tedious, it is essential; each of these behaviors must be over-learned to become habitual.

The only objective week-to-week measure you have of your behavior change is your weight change. Your weight loss will be maintained in proportion to the changes in your eating behaviors.

Maintenance is stressed, and the five-week Maintenance period is included in this program, because most people find that keeping weight off is the most difficult task of all. The Maintenance period is a way of letting you practice your new eating techniques in a semi-structured situation. Except for the Food Diary and the Daily Behavior Checklist, you were on your own, much as you will be when you finish this book. You will continue to receive a Daily Behavior Checklist each week from this point on, to help you focus on your new behaviors, and to give you points of reference in making them habitual.

Last lesson, five weeks ago, you were introduced to some general principles of problem solving, and you applied them to problem eating behaviors. Behavioral problem solving was divided into five parts:

1. ***Observation of Eating Behaviors.*** The Food Diaries you have filled out during the course have forced you to observe systematically your eating behaviors, including activities associated with eating.

2. ***Identification of Eating Problems.*** Everyone has a unique set of eating problems, which must eventually be dealt with, one at a time. During the problem-solving lesson you identified some of your unique eating problems.

3. ***Creative Problem Solving, or Brainstorming.*** It can be fun to make a list of as many solutions as possible for the problems you

identify. It was suggested that you start by listing them uncritically. Sometimes the most "far out" solutions work best.

4. ***Choosing the Best Plan.*** The next step was to decide which solution would best solve the problem and fit your lifestyle.

5. ***Building in Self-Evaluation and Feedback.*** If you don't evaluate your progress, you won't know when you are succeeding. You need a systematic method for evaluating each behavior change. The object of this exercise was to give you practice in defining and solving eating problems. By the end of this program, we would like you to feel confident planning and evaluating your own behavior change program, to feel confident as your own therapist.

Last lesson you analyzed your Food Diaries, and defined and worked out a specific behavioral solution for one of your eating problems. Your solution may have been as simple as eliminating a problem food (like peanut butter), or changing a cue (like not eating while talking on the phone), or introducing a new behavior (like swallowing between bites). The importance of a feedback or on-going evaluation of your program's success was stressed several times.

How Do You Stand Now?

- Did you define a problem? Yes_____ No_____

- Did you work out a solution and some form of feedback for self-evaluation? Yes_____ No_____

- Were you able to continue solving problems during the Maintenance period? Yes_____ No_____

- Do you feel competent to look at your own eating patterns to define specific problems, and to think of plans to change them? Yes_____ No_____ (If not, review Pages 82–85)

- What were some of the problems and solutions you worked on by yourself?

    1. _____

    2. _____

At this point, before new techniques are introduced, it is essential that you know where you stand, what your successes are in terms of behavior change, and what you need to review. Last week you kept a detailed Food Diary to help you answer these questions. Now we want you to fill out a Behavioral Analysis and Feedback Form at the end of this lesson, using the information from last week's Food Diary. Compare your eating behaviors during Week One, Week Four, and last week. This will give you some information about how well you have maintained your new behaviors, and it will also give you some clues about remaining problems you will need to work on. Is the pattern you see on the Behavioral Analysis and Feedback Form better, worse, or the same as the pattern five weeks ago?

Next, define a specific problem to work on for the coming week. Make a list of solutions, pick out the best solution, and finally devise some form of information feedback so you will know whether or not your problem solving is successful. Your materials for today include a Behavioral Prescription Sheet. After you analyze your Food Diary and define a problem, fill out the Behavioral Prescription Sheet. Include on the form the problem and the techniques you are going to work on this coming week.

Once again, the ultimate goal of this exercise is to make you an independent therapist, able to spot, define, and solve your own eating problems. You are reading this text to learn how to be an expert behavioral problem solver.

NEW TECHNIQUE: PRE-PLANNING WHAT YOU EAT.

Pre-planning is a technique many people find very useful in controlling their food intake. Unfortunately, it is a technique that almost everyone finds correspondingly difficult. Pre-planning is a way of thinking about food and the circumstances of eating. It is a technique designed to minimize the number of last-minute decisions about what to eat, and to diminish the effect of impulses to eat. It is a very effective way to deal with high-calorie foods before they reach your plate.

Pre-planning can become a very strong habit and can be especially useful when you are going to a party or out to eat at a restaurant. By thinking ahead you can plan strategies for these situations. If your strategies are thought out in advance, you will have a greater tendency to limit your intake than if you had not planned at all. Thinking ahead relieves you of the necessity for on-the-spot decisions.

When you pre-plan, you pre-decide when and what to eat. For example, you might decide that after a 10:00 a.m. snack of coffee and a banana you will not have anything else to eat until 12:30, when you have scheduled a bran muffin and a diet cola. If someone offers you a doughnut at 11:00, you will be more likely to turn it down if you have planned in advance not to eat at that time. This is especially true when your meals and snacks are committed to a written schedule. If that extra doughnut isn't on the plan, it is less tempting.

Another example would be pre-planning for dinner at a good restaurant. The idea would be to think ahead about the dinner, so you will know what you are going to eat when you get there. If you had planned for one cocktail, a fish entrée with a green salad, and sherbet, you would stand a better chance of not going along with the crowd and having three cocktails, soup, Beef Wellington, and a chocolate soufflé. If you enter the restaurant with a strategy, with preferences thought out in advance, you will be less influenced by impulse, and less tempted by high-calorie foods. When the second round of cocktails starts, you will still be working on your first one. When that extravagantly tempting menu is passed to you, you will be set to look at the fish section, and when dessert is proposed, you will be ready to order sherbet.

Because pre-planning involves a fundamental change in the way you think about food, this technique should be approached slowly, a step at a time. At first you should plan only one meal or snack a day. When you are able to pre-plan one meal and consistently follow the plan, increase your planning by one additional meal or snack a day. Keep increasing the amount of pre-planning until you are able to predict most of the food you will eat every day. The object of this exercise is to develop the skill of anticipating all of your eating behaviors in advance, and being able to pre-plan all of the food you eat. With the proper use of this technique, impulse eating will disappear.

The technique of pre-planning is divided into five steps. It is a set of activities that will develop into habit patterns over a long period of time if you conscientiously practice every day. As has been emphasized with all of the techniques in this book, you should not feel like you are in a race. Everyone develops the ability to pre-plan at a different rate. If you start feeling bad about the technique, or guilty because you are not able to do it completely, then you may be trying too hard. You should pre-plan fewer meals, and maintain that number until it feels comfortable to increase again.

These are the steps:

1. Set aside a time each day to think ahead and plan your food intake for that day. Include in your planning all food (and drink) that has significant caloric value.

2. Write down on your Food Diary the time, place, type of food, and amount of food you think you will eat during that day—make a menu. Be realistic about the amount of pre-planning you start with. Don't expect to pre-plan three meals a day until you have tried to pre-plan one meal a day.

   When you write down your pre-planned meal or meals on your Food Diary, use a pen or pencil of a different color than the one you are accustomed to using. After you have eaten your pre-planned meal, take out your regular pen and check your predictions.

Correct your pre-planned menu with your regular pen. As you become a better pre-planner, the number of two-colored entries will decrease. Again, wait until you are consistently successful in pre-planning one meal a day before you increase to two meals a day.

3. Try to *plan ahead* for eating out and for parties. Plan strategies: How many drinks will I have? What would really taste good besides Steak Diane? If I cannot avoid a high-calorie entrée, can I eat only part of it, or eat it over a long period of time?

4. If you find it hard to stick to pre-planning meals or snacks, one helpful technique is to *prepare your food* in the morning, label it for the time of consumption, and put it in a special place. When the time comes to snack or eat, it is ready. The tendency to go on and eat more, or to eat at the wrong time is minimized.

5. Pre-plan what you buy. A related and very important pre-planning technique applies to *shopping* for food. Write out a shopping list in advance, with specific brands of foods and the quantities you want to buy of each. Go to the store on a *full stomach* and try not to vary from the list. This technique will eliminate impulse buying. If you don't plan to buy snack foods, and manage to avoid them at the store, they will not be in the house to tempt you later.

Is This All Clear to You?

- Do you understand the concept of pre-planning? Yes_____
  No_____ (Page 146)

- Do you understand how to do the exercise, using two colored pens? Yes_____ No_____ (Page 147)

- When are you going to pre-plan, and for which meal or snack? Pre-planning Time: _____ Meal/Snack:_____

- Do you see how pre-planning can be used for parties, and social functions?

    1. For drinks, hors d'oeuvres, etc.

    2. For pre-planning portion size—and leaving some behind.

    3. For learning to eat more slowly—with control.

- Do any of the pre-planning techniques not make sense?

    1. Shopping from a list on a full stomach? Yes_____
       No_____

    2. Preparing snacks and meals in advance? Yes_____
       No_____

Turn now to the Daily Behavior Checklist for this week. You will see that pre-planning is listed with the other new behaviors. Each day indicate whether you did pre-plan a meal and how successful you were. If you *tried* (but were unsuccessful) rate yourself "1." If you got so far as to write your Diary in two colors, rate yourself "2." If you actually were able to *pre-plan accurately* at least *75 percent* of the time, rate yourself "3." Estimate your degree of success by how much of the pre-planned meal had to be corrected with another color ink after you ate the meal.

This is a difficult assignment. It takes time to pre-plan, and time is very hard to come by. Being able to pre-plan is a matter of establishing priorities. If this technique takes too much away from the rest of your life or interferes with your lifestyle, it may be necessary to approach it very gradually. If you do master it, you will find that pre-planning is one of the most powerful techniques for helping you to limit your food intake.

Many people find that pre-planning changes their entire outlook on food. There is no longer uncertainty about what they will eat. When all intake is pre-planned, there is no longer a temptation to snack. It is a very useful tool for decreasing total caloric intake and gaining a feeling of greater control over your eating behaviors.

HOMEWORK.

A. Lesson Six Food Diary.

B. Lesson Six Daily Behavior Checklist

C. Pre-planning of the Food Diaries for at least one meal a day.

D. Completion of a Behavioral Prescription Sheet, including some form of information feedback to let you know if your intervention was successful.

BEHAVIORAL ANALYSIS AND FEEDBACK FORM

TIME OF EATING

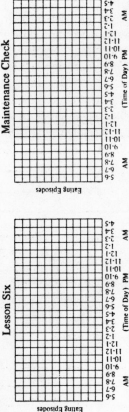

Indicate the time of day for each eating episode during the week by making a mark in the square above the appropriate time of day. Start with the bottom row of boxes. If you have a second eating episode during the week within that time range, indicate it by filling in the next box in that column. For example, if you had a snack at 10:30 am, you would fill in the first box in the time of day column labeled "10-11 am." If the next day, you had breakfast at 10:15 am, you would blacken in the next box up in that same column. If that same day, you had a snack at 10:50 am, you would indicate this by marking the third box in the same column. When you have entered an entire week's eating pattern in these boxes, you will have a graph which shows the distribution of your eating during the week.

MINUTES SPENT EATING

	Lesson Six		Maintenance Check	
	Meal	Snack	Meal	Snack
0-5 minutes......	_____	_____	_____	_____
5-10 minutes......	_____	_____	_____	_____
10-15 minutes......	_____	_____	_____	_____
15-20 minutes......	_____	_____	_____	_____
20-30 minutes......	_____	_____	_____	_____
over 30 minutes.....	_____	_____	_____	_____

Indicate the duration of *each* of your eating episodes by making a tally mark on the line under the appropriate heading — "meal" or "snack". For example, if breakfast took seven minutes, put a mark under the word "meal" on the line labeled "5-10 minutes." If you had a mid-afternoon snack that lasted 13 minutes, put a mark under "snack" on the line labeled "10-15 minutes." If you had six meals, each 5-10 minutes long, you would have six tallies (卌 I) in the meal column on the line marked 5-10 minutes.

(Adapted from and used by permission of Leonard S. Levitz, Ph.D., and Henry A. Jordan, M.D., University of Pennsylvania School of Medicine, "Analysis of Food Intake and Energy Expenditure," Copyright, 1973.)

BEHAVIORAL ANALYSIS AND FEEDBACK FORM
DEGREE OF HUNGER

	Lesson Six			Maintenance Check	
	Meal	Snack		Meal	Snack
0 – none	_____	_____	0 – none	_____	_____
1 – some	_____	_____	1 – some	_____	_____
2 – hungry	_____	_____	2 – hungry	_____	_____
3 – extreme	_____	_____	3 – extreme	_____	_____

Put a tally mark on the appropriate line to indicate the degree of hunger you felt at the beginning of every episode of eating during the week. For example, if you had a snack and were not hungry, put a mark under snack on the line labeled "none." If you felt like you were starving to death when you had dinner, put a mark under "meal" on the line labeled "extreme." (Note: Use the same numbers that appear on your Week One Food Diary.)

BODY POSITION WHILE EATING

	Lesson Six			Maintenance Check	
	Meal	Snack		Meal	Snack
Walking	_____	_____	Walking	_____	_____
Standing	_____	_____	Standing	_____	_____
Sitting	_____	_____	Sitting	_____	_____
Lying Down	_____	_____	Lying Down	_____	_____

Put a tally mark on the appropriate line to indicate your body position during each episode of eating for the week. For example, if you had a snack while walking around the grocery store, put a mark under "snack" on the line labeled "walking." If you ate dinner lying in bed watching television, put a mark under "meal" on the line labeled "lying down."

ACTIVITIES WHILE EATING

	Lesson Six		Maintenance Check	
	Meal	Snack	Meal	Snack
None: only eating	_____	_____	_____	_____
Talking	_____	_____	_____	_____
Listening to music or radio	_____	_____	_____	_____
Reading a book or paper	_____	_____	_____	_____
Watching television	_____	_____	_____	_____
Cooking-working in kitchen	_____	_____	_____	_____
Working-studying	_____	_____	_____	_____
Other	_____	_____	_____	_____

Put a tally mark on the appropriate line to indicate activities that are associated with your episodes of eating. For example, if you ate lunch while working at your desk, put a mark under "meal" on the line labeled "working." If you had a snack while preparing dinner, put a mark under the "snack" column on the line labeled "cooking."

(Adapted from and used by permission of Leonard S. Levitz, Ph.D., and Henry A. Jordan, M.D., University of Pennsylvania School of Medicine, "Analysis of Food Intake and Energy Expenditure," Copyright, 1973.)

FOOD DIARY – Lesson Six

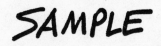

Day of Week __MONDAY__   Name__C. B. T.__

Time	Minutes Spent Eating	M/S	H	Food Type & Quantity	Individual Techniques *EAT SNACKS AT DESIGNATION PLACE*
6:00					
7:20 - 7:30	10 MIN	M	0	COFFEE, CEREAL	YES ★
8:15 - 8:20	5 MIN	S	0	COFFEE, DONUT	NO
11:00					
3:30 - 3:40	10 MIN	M	3	HAMBURG.	YES ★
4:00					
6:00 - 7:00	1 HR	M	2	BEEF TV DINNER ICE CREAM	YES ★
9:00					
10:30 - 10:45	15 MIN	S	0	ICE CREAM	YES ★

FOOD DIARY – Lesson Six

Day of Week _____   Name_____

Time	Minutes Spent Eating	M/S	H	Food Type & Quantity	Individual Techniques
6:00					
11:00					
4:00					
9:00					

FOOD DIARY – Lesson Six

Day of Week _____   Name_____

Time	Minutes Spent Eating	M/S	H	Food Type & Quantity	Individual Techniques
6:00					
11:00					
4:00					
9:00					

FOOD DIARY – Lesson Six

Day of Week _____   Name_____

Time	Minutes Spent Eating	M/S	H	Food Type & Quantity	Individual Techniques
6:00					
11:00					
4:00					
9:00					

FOOD DIARY -- Lesson Six

Day of Week _____   Name_____

Time	Minutes Spent Eating	M/S	H	Food Type & Quantity	Individual Techniques
6:00					
11:00					
4:00					
9:00					

FOOD DIARY – Lesson Six

Day of Week _____ Name _____

Time	Minutes Spent Eating	M/S	H	Food Type & Quantity	Individual Techniques
6:00					
11:00					
4:00					
9:00					

FOOD DIARY – Lesson Six

Day of Week _____   Name_____

Time	Minutes Spent Eating	M/S	H	Food Type & Quantity	Individual Techniques
6:00					
11:00					
4:00					
9:00					

FOOD DIARY – Lesson Six

Day of Week _____   Name_____

Time	Minutes Spent Eating	M/S	H	Food Type & Quantity	Individual Techniques
6:00					
11:00					
4:00					
9:00					

DAILY BEHAVIOR CHECKLIST – Lesson Six

Points: Most of the time, or yes = 3
          Sometimes   = 2
          Not at all, or no   = 1

Days of the Week

	1	2	3	4	5	6	7
1. *Daily Checklist* a. Morning Review							
b. Evening scoring							
2. *Food Diary* a. Recording my food							
3. *Cue Elimination* a. Designated eating place							
b. Only eating when eating							
c. Food out of sight							
4. *Eating Delay* a. Utensils down between mouthfuls							
b. Swallowing each forkful before adding the next							
c. Enjoying the meal							
5. *Behavior Chains* a. Break a behavior chain							
b. Substitute an activity for eating							
6. *Pre-planning* a. Pre-plan one or more meals or snacks							
7. *Becoming Your Own Therapist* a. Individual problem solving or working on individual problem							
DAILY TOTALS							

Total Points for the Week _____   Weight _____

BEHAVIORAL PRESCRIPTION SHEET —

Name _____

Partner _____

Problem _____

_____

_____

_____

Solutions _____

_____

_____

_____

_____

_____

_____

_____

_____

_____

Plan _____

_____

_____

_____

_____

_____

Feedback _____

_____

_____

Consultation _____

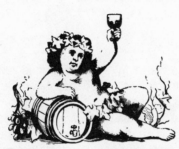

Lesson Seven

Cue Elimination, Part Two And Energy Use, Part One

WEIGH-IN AND HOMEWORK.

Weigh yourself and graph your weight change.

Check your homework.

—Is your Lesson Six Food Diary complete? Yes_____
No_____

—Have you included pre-planning on your Food Diary?
Yes_____ No_____

—Is your Daily Behavior Checklist for Lesson Six filled in?
Yes_____ No_____

—Is your individual problem solving completed? Yes_____
No_____

Give yourself credit for your homework.

163

REVIEW: MAINTENANCE AND
THE BEHAVIOR CHECKLIST.

The behavior therapies emphasize Maintenance of behaviors once they have been established. The Daily Behavior Checklist is a tool to help improve the odds of successful Maintenance. For the next four weeks fill in the checklist every day, and try to improve your score as the weeks progress. At the end of the text you will have a final Behavior Checklist. When you are confident your new eating skills are habitual, the checklist can be eliminated. When you feel a need to brush up on your new habits, reintroduce the checklist for a few weeks (if necessary, making additional copies for yourself). Periodic practice is one way to assure successful Maintenance.

Pre-planning.

The technique of pre-planning was introduced last week. A good way to increase the probability that your behavior will be different in the future is to make definite plans and commit yourself to a course of action in advance. You will be more likely to limit your food intake if you plan ahead to eat specific foods at pre-selected times and places. It's much more effective than simply saying to yourself, "I'm going to be more careful about what I eat."

Self-instruction and expectation play a large part in how hungry you are during the day. If each meal and snack is scheduled, and you stick to the schedule long enough, the question of whether or not you are hungry will not cross your mind when food is not on your schedule—for example, when candy is served unexpectedly at the office, or when you pass a vending machine or a bakery. Regardless of the feeling, you won't eat because you haven't planned for it; and the strength of the stimulus telling you to eat will be weakened each time you ignore it.

Pre-planning is a time-consuming project at first. Like the Food Diary, it takes much less time after you've practiced doing it. In fact, the time used thinking about filling it out may be the most time-consuming and anxiety-provoking part of the exercise. Pre-planning is a technique that can be approached in steps. Pre-plan one meal a day, then add a second meal, or a snack, and continue until the whole day's food intake is planned in advance. For some people, for example those who plan meals for a family, this technique will be easy. For others it may take a month or more before the ability to plan each meal in advance becomes a habit.

Pre-planning can be divided into a series of steps: First, designate a time each day to think ahead and plan meals and snacks, at first only one meal or snack for each day. Second, actually write down these plans in your Food Diary. Third, correct your pre-planned meals with a different colored pen after you eat a meal. These different colored notations emphasize the difference between the amount and type of food you planned and the food you actually ate. If snacks are difficult to plan, it might be easier to prepare them in advance, label them for a specific time, and eat them when you planned to snack.

Another use of pre-planning is at parties or when you go out to dinner. If you anticipate an unavoidable large meal, you can plan to decrease your food intake earlier in the day to make up for a planned calorie excess. You can also plan strategies for parties: how many drinks you will have, how many hors d'oeuvres, how much cake you will have for dessert, etc.

How Did This Go?

- Do you have any questions about the theory, definition, or reason for pre-planning? Yes_____ No_____ (Page 146)

- Do you have any questions about how the pre-planning should be done? Yes_____ No_____ (Page 147)

- Were you able to pre-plan a restaurant meal and actually carry out your contingency plan? Yes_____ No_____

- Did you notice any changes in your eating pattern, particularly with respect to impulse eating? Yes_____ No_____

It is all right to switch equal foods like peas and beans, or simply to provide for a type of food when you will be eating in a restaurant. In pre-planning the spirit is more important than the letter of the theory.

The final point in pre-planning was very important: changing your food-buying behavior by pre-planning when you will shop and what you will buy. When you shop for food, make a shopping list which includes everything you are going to buy, very specifically listed by brand name and quantity. Go to the store on a full stomach to avoid impulse buying, and try not to vary from your shopping list. This will help you avoid buying snack foods and products which contain only empty calories. Food that is not bought and is not within easy reach will not be eaten.

Do You Feel You Made Progress?

- Did you go shopping on a full stomach? Yes_____ No_____

- Did you notice a change in your attraction to impulse foods at the market? Yes_____ No_____

- Were you able to pre-plan and shop from a list? Yes_____ No_____

CUE ELIMINATION: PART TWO
(ABOUT THOSE STARVING ARMENIANS).

In the first discussion of cue elimination you were told that overweight people tend to be controlled more by environmental stimuli than thin people. They tend to be more sensitive to the smell and sight of food, and places associated with food, than their thin friends. At that time several methods of eliminating cues (or environmental reminders) that often lead to inappropriate eating were introduced. These were:

1. Eat only at a Designated Appropriate Eating Place.
2. Change your habitual eating place at the table.
3. When you are eating, only eat—no other activities.
4. Work to reduce visual food cues: remove food from all places in the house other than appropriate storage areas. Store food in opaque containers to keep it out of sight.
5. Have alternate foods available to replace high impulse or "junk" foods.
6. Do not leave serving dishes on the table.

All of these exercises helped reduce the potency of food cues in your environment. These six rules, if followed carefully, will affect almost all inappropriate eating, and will help you build a new set of responses to former food cues. For example, by now you are probably watching the 6:00 news for information instead of for permission to eat.

All of the cue elimination exercises in lesson 3 involved stimuli that were physically removed from food. Today you will receive six additional exercises that will help eliminate cues more closely associated with the act of eating. These exercises appear deceptively simple, and you may find that you are not able to do all of them immediately. The more of them you can master, the higher the probability of your success in losing weight. Some of the techniques may not be applicable at all times; for example, using smaller plates when you are at a restaurant. However, most people are able to use these cue elimination techniques most of the time without difficulty.

1. **Smaller plates.** Research has shown that the size of the plate your food is served on has a large influence on how you perceive the amount of food you are eating, and consequently, how full you feel after the meal. Even though you know that the size of the plate does not make any difference—a spoonful of potatoes is basically a spoonful of potatoes—it seems like more food when it is served on a smaller plate. A psychology experiment demon-

strated that 70 percent of the people in a weight reduction program were more satisfied with less food when it was served on a salad plate than when it was served on a dinner plate.[4] This week we would like you to try eating from smaller plates; try to make them a part of your daily routine.

2. **Set Some Aside.**   All of us have been strongly conditioned to eat everything on our plates, and to feel guilty when we leave some behind. Whether for economy, aesthetics, or because of all the starving children in Armenia, China, or elsewhere, almost everyone has been taught this lesson. Not wasting food is usually a very well learned irrational idea. The implicit belief is that if we finish our meals and eat everything on our plate, it will benefit someone else. The unfortunate corollary to this is, "If I do not finish everything on my plate, somehow I am bad."

   One could consider the history of this concept and how possibly it evolved during times of famine. But it would serve no purpose; many of us are stuck with it, whatever its origin. It is, of course, a very false economy. It leads to eating more than we need, because we feel we must finish and not leave food to be thrown away.

   The second assignment for today is to start breaking this habit, to begin to free yourself of the compulsion to eat everything you are served. To accomplish this, leave food behind at each meal. Start out slowly: one pea, a spoonful of potatoes, or a crust of bread from your sandwich. It may be necessary to set the leftover food aside at the start of the meal and cover it with plastic wrap so you won't forget to leave it behind. Or, at the other end of the meal, you may find it necessary to put the leftover food in the garbage immediately, to prevent yourself from eating it. (This technique can be used later for eliminating problem foods and reducing portion size.) For today, concentrate on leaving some food on your plate after every meal.

3. **Seconds.**   For those eating large portions, especially at dinner, divide the food you would normally serve yourself into two servings, and go back for seconds when you finish the first half. This introduces a delay, and hopefully a cognitive or thinking step in the middle of the meal, e.g., "Do I really want seconds or thirds?" It has the added advantage of keeping the second half of the meal warm and more enjoyable when you do eat it. Don't forget to leave some of each portion behind.

4. **Throw Away.**   Throw away any food left on your plate immediately after the meal. Put scraps down the disposal, in the garbage can,

or feed them to the cat. In this way they won't linger around to be nibbled on later in the evening or the next afternoon. If you do keep something, like a chicken wing or a serving of peas, pre-plan it into a snack for the next day or as part of lunch. Put it in an opaque container and label it with its specific pre-planned use, e.g., "John's Lunch." Don't let food hang around the house loose and uncommitted! It will reach out and cue you to eat.

5. **Ask for Food.** Never accept food from another person unless you ask for it. Make each encounter with food a voluntary one. In restaurants, take the initiative—ask the server not to bring potatoes, or to take away the bread. If it is not on the table, you won't nibble on it while you wait for your meal.

6. **Minimize Contact.** Try to arrange your food contacts in ways that minimize the chances for impulse eating. For example, when you fix yourself a sandwich for lunch, put away the bread, butter, and jelly, and clean up the mess before you eat your sandwich. This will greatly reduce the likelihood that you will make a second sandwich. Food out of sight is often food out of mind.

Do You Understand the Need for This Second Set of Cue Elimination Exercises?

These exercises deal with cues inherent in the act of eating—the previous elimination exercises dealt with more general environmental cues. Every time you sit down to eat, think of the starving Armenians and follow these six steps: (1) use smaller plates, (2) leave some food behind, (3) split large meals into several portions, (4) throw leftovers away or pre-plan them for a specific use, (5) ask for food when you want it, and (6) organize your environment to minimize chances for impulse eating.

The old cue elimination exercises are still valid. The less conspicuous food is, and the less you respond to environmental stimuli that remind you to eat, the better your eating habits will become.

ENERGY: PART ONE (THERE IS NO CRISIS, JUST A CONTINUING PROBLEM).

(You will need a pedometer for this and subsequent lessons. They can be purchased at sporting goods, variety, and specialty stores.)

A simple equation can be written for how to gain and lose weight. This equation holds true for everyone—and the entire animal kingdom:

ENERGY IN (food) = ENERGY USED (activity) + STORAGE (fat)

So far you have worked on the "energy in" side of the equation, by modifying your intake and causing a decrease in the amount of energy consumed. This has shifted the balance of the equation and has allowed some of your storage energy (fat) to be burned up. For the next two weeks you will be working on the other side of the equation—"energy used," or activity. To understand this topic most meaningfully, you will have to think in terms of calories. However, the calories you are concerned with in this lesson are those used up rather than those eaten.

This week we want to introduce the topic of energy use and have you make some observations about your activity. Next lesson we will talk more about energy use and introduce some techniques to increase energy expenditure (without calisthenics).

Exercise is one of the hardest behaviors to build into one's routine. Lying on the couch or sitting in front of television can be very pleasant compared to moving about, especially if you're overweight and out of shape. If your only activity is watching television, it may be of some comfort to know that your Basal Metabolic Rate, the amount of energy you consume while you are resting, increases 20 percent if you sit rather than lie down to watch T-V; it increases even more if you stand rather than sit, but not many people like to stand while they watch T-V.

It is commonly believed that exercise doesn't play much of a role in losing weight. After all, even jogging only burns up ten Calories per minute. Actually an increased expenditure of energy is very important to weight loss programs. Regular exercise should increase the rate of weight loss, and for many people who have reached a plateau on a weight loss program, exercise can reestablish their downward trend.

Contrary to popular belief, expending more energy usually does not lead to an increase in appetite. Studies have shown that food intake actually decreases when the average person increases his or her level of physical activity.[5] Because of this, exercise can actually contribute to food restriction in weight reduction programs. This week you will analyze some of your activities and begin to think about their caloric "worth." Remember that an extra 250 Calories burned each day is equal to one-half pound of weight loss a week, or 26 pounds lost each year, with no change in food intake.

During the coming week, you will collect two types of data to give yourself a baseline or starting point for next week's lesson:

1. Record (on the Daily Activity Sheet at the end of this lesson) the number of minutes you spend in physical activity *in addition* to the activity of your daily routine. Examples of extra activities would be gardening, golfing, running, swimming, and moving furniture. Next week you will convert these minutes of exercise to their caloric equivalent to help you make some changes that will burn up extra calories. (Do not fill in the spaces marked for "Calories." You will do that next lesson.)

2. Keep track of the number of miles you walk each day. Wear your pedometer and record on the Daily Activity Sheet the miles that register on the dial at the end of each day.

The pedometer converts the up and down motion of your body when you walk, to a measure of distance. (Inside the pedometer is a small pendulum that moves up and down with each step you take. These movements of the pendulum are translated by gears into a series of small movements of the needle on the face of the pedometer. The farther you walk, the more up and down movements, and the more distance registered on the dial.)

To use the pedometer accurately, you must program it for the length of your stride. This allows the device to calculate the distance you have traveled on the basis of your number of steps and the average length of each step. Your stride is determined by counting the number of steps you make in a standard distance, and dividing this into the distance walked. For example, if you take 50 steps when you walk a distance of 100 feet, the length of your stride is two feet (100 feet divided by 50 steps = 2 feet per step).

Set the pedometer for the length of your stride. Every evening write down the number of miles you have walked during the day. After you write down your mileage, turn the meter back to zero to start the next day's recording.

Do not try to compute calories at this point. Next week you will calculate your present activity level, and you will be given some strategies to help you increase your daily energy expenditure.

Is This All Clear?

- Do you understand the energy equation and terms used in it? Yes_____ No_____ (Pages 168, 169)

- Be sure you understand the assignment and how to use the pedometer before you begin this week's assignment. If necessary, ask someone at a sport shop to help you adjust it. Once it is adjusted, don't change it.

HOMEWORK.

A. Complete the Lesson Seven Food Diary.

B. Continue pre-planning at least one meal or snack a day. If this has become comfortable, increase by a meal or snack each day.

C. Fill in your Daily Behavior Checklist every day. Some of the new cue elimination exercises are on the checklist for this week.

D. Write down the miles you walk each day, as well as the number of minutes spent in non-routine exercise during the next week on the Daily Activity Sheet.

FOOD DIARY – Lesson Seven

Day of Week_____   Name_____

Time	M/S	Location	Activity While Eating	Food Type and Quantity
6:00				
11:00				
4:00				
9:00				

FOOD DIARY – Lesson Seven

Day of Week_____   Name_____

Time	M/S	Location	Activity While Eating	Food Type and Quantity
6:00				
11:00				
4·00				
9:00				

FOOD DIARY – Lesson Seven

Day of Week_____   Name _____

Time	M/S	Location	Activity While Eating	Food Type and Quantity
6:00				
11:00				
4:00				
9:00				

FOOD DIARY — Lesson Seven

Day of Week_____   Name_____

Time	M/S	Location	Activity While Eating	Food Type and Quantity
6:00				
11:00				
4:00				
9:00				

FOOD DIARY -- Lesson Seven

Day of Week_____   Name_____

Time	M/S	Location	Activity While Eating	Food Type and Quantity
6:00				
11:00				
4:00				
9:00				

FOOD DIARY – Lesson Seven

Day of Week_____   Name_____

Time	M/S	Location	Activity While Eating	Food Type and Quantity
6:00				
11:00				
4:00				
9:00				

FOOD DIARY – Lesson Seven

Day of Week_____   Name_____

Time	M/S	Location	Activity While Eating	Food Type and Quantity
6:00				
11:00				
4:00				
9:00				

DAILY BEHAVIOR CHECKLIST – Lesson Seven

Points: Most of the time, or yes **= 3**
        Sometimes   **= 2**
        Not at all, or no   **= 1**

				Days			
	1	2	3	4	5	6	7
1. *Daily Checklist* a. Morning Review							
b. Evening Scoring							
2. *Food Diary* a. Recording my food							
3. *Cue Elimination – I* a. Designated eating place							
b. Only eating when eating							

4. *Eating Delay*
  a. Swallow each forkful before
    adding the next							

5. *Behavior Chains*
  a. Substitute an activity for
    eating							

6. *Pre-planning*
  a. Pre-plan one or more meals or
    snacks							

b. Shop on a full stomach							

7. *Cue Elimination – II*
  a. Use smaller plates when
    possible							

b. Leave food behind on the plate							
c. Split large meals into seconds							
d. Throw away or commit leftovers							
e. Don't accept food from others							
f. Minimize your contact with food.							
Daily Totals							

Total Points for the Week _____   Weight _____

DAILY ACTIVITY SHEET

SAMPLE

(Fill in miles per day walked and minutes of exercise or extra activities)

	Monday		Tuesday		Wednesday		Thursday		Friday		Saturday		Sunday	
	Miles	Calories	Miles	Calories	Miles	Calories	Miles	Calories	Miles	Calories	Miles	Calories	Miles	Calories
Miles Walked	2½	350	3	420	2	286	3½	490	4	560	2	280	2½	315
Activity or Exercise	Mins.	Calories	Mins.	Calories	Mins.	Calories	Mins.	Calories	Mins.	Calories	Mins.	Calories	Mins.	Calories
BOWLING (ACTUAL ACTIVITY)			40	360										
GARDENING											30	141		
MOW LAWN (POWER)											40	212		
SWIMMING													20	126

DAILY ACTIVITY SHEET

(Fill in miles per day walked and minutes of exercise or extra activities)

		Monday		Tuesday		Wednesday		Thursday		Friday		Saturday		Sunday	
		Miles	Calories	Miles	Calories	Miles	Calories	Miles	Calories	Miles	Calories	Miles	Calories	Miles	Calories
Miles Walked															
Activity or Exercise	Mins.	Calories	Mins.	Calories	Mins.	Calories	Mins.	Calories	Mins.	Calories	Mins.	Calories	Mins.	Calories	

Copyright 1975,
Bull Publishing Co.

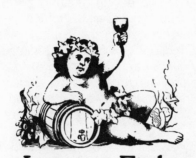

Lesson Eight

Energy Use, Part Two

WEIGH-IN AND HOMEWORK.

Weigh yourself, record your weight on the Master Data Sheet and graph your weight change.

Homework:

—Is your Lesson Seven Food Diary complete? Yes_____ No_____

—Is your pre-planning written on the Food Diary? Yes_____ No_____

—Is your Daily Behavior Checklist for Lesson Seven up to date? Yes_____ No_____

—Are the minutes of exercise (by category) and miles walked recorded on your Daily Activity Sheet? Yes_____ No_____

REVIEW: CUE ELIMINATION, PART TWO.

Last lesson's cue elimination exercises were designed to change your response to cues common in eating and food-related activities. In many ways these are harder cues to ignore than more remote environmental stimuli like television and vending machines. Food-related cues are present every time you sit down to eat.

The use of smaller plates has been found by many to be very effective in eliminating a strong cue related to meal size; the smaller plates take advantage of a tendency everyone has to judge the size of a meal by how well it fills the plate.

You were asked to stop feeding the starving Armenian inside yourself and to leave some food on your plate after each meal. The effect of this exercise is to eliminate the feeling that a meal ends when the plate is clean. Unfortunately, most of us were taught this habit as children, and find it is surprisingly difficult to break.

Splitting large portions in half and going back for the second half is a way of introducing both a delay and a thinking break into the meal. By the time you decide to have the second part of the meal, you may no longer want it.

Throwing away excess food, or labeling it for its future use, eliminates the cue to eat that is usually associated with leftovers. This technique can provide an easy way of freeing yourself from an old snacking habit.

The final two cue elimination techniques were: never accept food from others—always ask for what you want, whether it is at home or in a restaurant; and minimize contact with food—the easiest way is to clean up the mess you make preparing food before you eat what you have prepared. (In the process of getting all the food out again you will think twice about that second sandwich or third piece of toast and jam in the morning.)

WAS LAST WEEK'S LESSON
EASY OR DIFFICULT?

- Do you have any questions about last week's cue elimination exercises? Yes_____ No_____

- Did you try smaller plates? Yes_____ No_____

- Were you able to leave food behind on your plate? Yes_____ No_____ Did it change the feeling you should clean up your plate? Yes_____ No_____ (It will vanish with time.)

- Were you able to deal successfully with leftovers—either throwing them away immediately, feeding them to the cat or disposal, or

pre-planning and labeling them for a specific use? Yes_____
No_____

Leaving food behind can control the size of a meal, at home or
at a party—when they pass the hors d'oeuvres, only eat half of one, leave
some of your drink behind in the glass, etc. Each of the cue elimination
techniques can be used in a variety of eating situations.

ENERGY: PART TWO
(THE CONTINUATION OF A CRISIS).

Last week we introduced the idea of an energy balance between calories
consumed and calories burned up. An equation can be written:

ENERGY IN (food) = ENERGY USED (activity) + STORAGE (fat)

or,

STORAGE (fat) = ENERGY IN (food) − ENERGY USED (activity)

This is a simplified form of one of the fundamental laws that governs
the universe, the Second Law of Thermodynamics. There are no exceptions
to this law, for man or beast.

During the first seven lessons, this program concentrated on the
"ENERGY IN" side of the equation. The net effect of your work to date
has diminished "ENERGY IN," by slowing your eating to allow you to
feel satiety or fullness, by eliminating cues to inappropriate eating, by
avoiding snacks with substitution techniques, and by changing your self-
instructions about impulse eating (through pre-planning). By reducing the
"ENERGY IN" side of the equation, you tipped the balance towards the
"ENERGY USED" side. You haven't taken in as much energy, and as
a result some of your stored energy or fat has been burned up.

Last week you learned that the "ENERGY USED" side of the equation is very important, and that it can act very effectively along with reduced
food intake to cause weight loss. Often an increase in exercise will reestablish the downward trend for individuals who have reached a plateau where
they feel stymied about continued weight loss. For others a modest addition
of exercise to their weight control program can accelerate their rate of
weight loss.

Most people are not aware of the amount of exercise they get each
day, or its effect on their weight. One study of obese housewives found
that they spent more of their time in light activities such as sleeping, sitting,
and watching television than a matched group of thin women. The thin
subjects used one sixth more energy during the day than the overweight
women, despite the fact that obese people use more calories per movement
because of the extra work involved in moving their extra weight.[6]

Common sense tells us that if we exercise more we will become more hungry. This is true within a "natural" range of activities for most animals, including humans. But in a way we no longer live in a "natural" state. In the natural state, or even 50 years ago in our civilized society, people got more exercise than they do today. The average American now spends much of his life sitting, or in equally mild activity. We are the most efficient people in the history of the world—and we show it!

We are no longer operating in our "natural" activity range, and we are suffering from the same phenomenon that ranchers exploit when they put cattle in a feedlot. When penned up with excess food available, a steer eats more, becomes fat and less mobile, exercises less, gains weight, eats more, etc. It is a vicious cycle. Several studies have shown that humans who adopt a sedentary life increase their food intake like the steers in the feedlot.[7] Conversely, when sedentary desk-bound people become more active—for example, when they change to a more active job—they eat less, and they lose weight.

Six bonuses can be gained by working on the "ENERGY USED" (or increased activity) side of the energy equation:

1. If you incorporate exercise into your daily routine, a higher proportion of the weight you lose will come from fat deposits, the energy your body has stored as fat.

2. Some form of exertion or activity added to a dull routine can relieve some of the boredom (or blues) that frequently stimulates eating.

3. Strenuous exercise has a specific effect on appetite, particularly if you exercise hard before a meal. Frequently it will markedly decrease your appetite.

4. As you lose weight, your body will regain a thin athletic shape.

5. Your body tone will improve, and your cardiovascular system will regain its ability to respond rapidly to stress and exercise.

6. You will enjoy life more.

Before we go too far with a discussion of expending more energy by increasing activity, we need to look at some basic calculations and arrive at a feeling for what exercise calories mean—where all of that energy goes.

1. Energy is necessary to keep your body alive, to maintain vital functions: heart beat, breathing, body temperature, muscle tone, etc. The actual amount needed, the Basal Metabolic Rate (BMR), is affected by many factors: You burn more energy, or have a higher BMR, with excess weight, increased surface area, fevers (14 percent

elevation in BMR for each degree centigrade of fever), pregnancy, thyroid disease, and anxiety. Metabolic rates and food requirements are lower in old people, Chinese, Indians, individuals who are starved for a long time, and depressed patients. The BMR is lower in women than in men. But regardless of an individual's metabolic rate, the laws of thermodynamics and the Energy Equation still hold true. A low BMR simply means you will have to lower your food intake below the point where people with a higher metabolic rate experience a weight loss; you need less energy (food) to stay at a constant weight, and you need less to lose weight.

2. Energy is used to digest food. Digesting proteins requires more calories than digesting fats, but the total amount of energy consumed in the digestion is low, regardless of food type—less than seven percent of your total energy intake. (And claims that all protein calories are burned up in digestion are nonsense.)

3. All physical activity uses up energy. Sitting increases energy expenditure over lying down, and standing increases it even more—of course, physical activity increases it further.

4. Energy is stored when you consume more than you burn. The storage is in high energy deposits of fat.

How many calories do you need each day and how many calories should you eat if you want to lose weight? The simplest approximation is often found in tables like the one on p. 188. This data is for the "average-weight" American. Occupation, activity level, body size, and the factors influencing Basal Metabolic Rate are *not* allowed for in this table.

Another (very rough) way to estimate your Maintenance caloric requirement is to multiply your body weight by 15. For example, if you weigh 200 pounds, the approximate number of calories needed to maintain your body weight is 3000 Calories per day. (200 × 15 = 3000 Calories.) To lose weight your caloric intake must be below this figure. If you are relatively inactive, your caloric need for weight maintenance will probably be significantly below this figure.

Remember, every table and calorie calculation is *approximate*. The only way to determine *your* need is to progressively decrease your intake until you are steadily losing weight. Remember too, as your weight drops, your daily caloric need also drops—there is less of you to feed.

One pound of body fat is equal to an excess intake of 3500 Calories. Thus a daily reduction of 500 Calories below your daily caloric needs for maintenance of body weight will cause you to lose one pound a week. (500 Calories × 7 days = 3500 Calories.)

There are many refinements and correction factors that would have to be provided for if the calculation were to accurately predict exactly

Figure 8-1
Recommended Daily Dietary Allowances, Food and Nutrition Board, National Research Council, National Academy of Sciences.

	Age[b] (years) From Up to	Weight (lbs)	Height (in.)	Calories
Infants	0–1/6	9	22	kg × 35
	1/6–1/2	15	25	kg × 50
	1/2–1	20	28	kg × 45.5
Children	1–2	26	32	1,000
	2–3	31	36	1,250
	3–4	35	39	1,400
	4–6	42	43	1,600
	6–8	51	48	2,000
	8–10	62	52	2,200
Males	10–12	77	55	2,500
	12–14	95	59	2,700
	14–18	130	67	3,000
	18–22	147	69	2,800
	22–35	154	69	2,800
	35–55	154	68	2,600
	55–75+	154	67	2,400
Females	10–12	77	56	2,250
	12–14	97	61	2,300
	14–16	114	62	2,400
	16–18	119	63	2,300
	18–22	128	64	2,000
	22–35	128	64	2,000
	35–55	128	63	1,850
	55–75+	128	62	1,700
Pregnancy				+200
Lactation				+1,000

how much a pound of *your* weight is worth in calories. However, even the best figures are not entirely accurate, and they cannot be calculated without extensive laboratory tests. These rough guides have a potential error of up to 25 percent, but they are close enough to allow us to meaningfully discuss the energy values of different activities.

The absolute values for caloric expenditure you calculate today will be interesting. But they are only important if you are able to take advantage of what you learn to change both your energy intake and your energy expenditure.

Is This Clear So Far?

- Do you have any questions about the theory of energy balance or the Energy Equation? Yes_____ No_____ (Pages 168–170)

- Do you understand where the energy goes that you consume in the form of food? Yes_____ No_____

- Did you get confused by the discussion of how to calculate the number of calories you need each day to maintain your current weight? Yes_____ No_____ (Page 187)

Keep in mind the fact that one pound of fat is the equivalent of 3500 Calories—3500 taken in *beyond* the amount needed to maintain your body weight if you are to gain a pound; and 3500 Calories burned off *beyond* what is taken in if you are to lose a pound.

The lesson today deals with a sort of heresy—how to systematically *waste* energy. We want you to learn how to expend more effort and burn up more calories in the course of your routine daily activities. The quickest way to burn up calories is to make large, fast movements, using as many large muscles as possible. This is why sports like swimming, tennis, cycling, and jogging are good exercise. However, activities like these are not always possible, available, appropriate, or in your price range. And you may find them unpleasant. If you are like most people, you won't stick with anything for long if it is unpleasant. At least at the start, less strenuous increases will probably be more effective.

There are two ways to increase your energy expenditure:

1. Increase your normal activities by becoming less efficient. Ask yourself the following question before you expend a single Calorie: "Is this the most energetic or wasteful way I can do this?" When possible, sit instead of lie, stand instead of sit, take stairs instead of elevators, and walk instead of ride, etc.

2. Introduce specific exercises, or increased activity, into your daily schedule.

   In the next two or three weeks you should find that you can easily increase your energy expenditure by 250 Calories a day, by being both wasteful and energetic. In fact, some people can jump right in and add 250 extra Calories of daily activity the first week. However, for most people, this, like all changes, will be difficult at first, and should probably be approached in steps of 50–100 Calories per day each week. This will be easy if you are able to start a systematic daily exercise program.

   Remember, when you are able to expend 250 Calories worth of extra exercise every day, you will be rewarded with an extra half pound of weight loss each week (or 26 extra pounds in a year).

ASSIGNMENT.

First, increase your daily activity by becoming less efficient. To give yourself information about your increase in activity continue to wear your pedometer and record the number of miles you walk each day. During the coming week try to walk 50 percent more miles each day than last week. For example, if you are currently walking three miles a day, increase your mileage to four and a half miles next week. (3 miles + 1½ miles =

4½ miles.) The following are some ways to build an increase in walking into your everyday routine:

1. Answer the phone farthest away (but still close enough to get it before the ringing stops). If you have to get up to answer it, good; that is the best part. The phone company estimates that an extension phone saves you 70 miles a year of walking.[8] This is equivalent to 20 pounds in ten years.

2. Use the farthest bathroom at home and at work.

3. Park the car at the far end of the parking lot or an extra block from the store or your appointment. Choose the long way of walking places. (Leave a little early so you get there on time.) You will eventually enjoy these walks as a brief "time out."

4. Use stairs instead of elevators.

5. Stand as much as possible.

6. Walk rather than drive whenever possible.

7. Meet the bus at the next station down the line.

Be creative about ways to expend more energy. Extra activity becomes more enjoyable with time, practice, and mastery. Just as lethargy can become a habit, so can activity.

Do These Ideas Get You Thinking About Extra Activity?

• Do you see how to use these hints to increase your walking next week? Yes_____ No_____

• Can you think of additional ways to walk farther during the day?

1. _____

2. _____

3. _____

Remember to record your mileage at the end of each day.

The second part of today's assignment is to increase the calories you expend in exercise. The easiest way to do this is to follow these guidelines:

1. Choose something you like to do, either a sport or more routine activity. Exercise does not have to be strenuous—some examples are gardening, easy jogging, and walking around the block.

2. Be sensible; start slowly and avoid strains that can catapult you back to a sitting (or lying) position.

3. Try to plan exercise ahead and arrange a partner, for company and so that the temptation to avoid your exercise at the last moment is reduced. Most people find it easier to exercise if they are with someone else, whether it is jogging or sex.

4. Choose active sports.

Record the number of minutes you spend exercising or in special activities on your Daily Activity Sheet. The materials for this lesson include a list of the caloric values of various activities. Make a rough estimate of the number of calories you spend each day in physical activity other than walking, and try to increase it week by week. The more you burn up, the faster you will lose. Make exercise one of your new habits—it's worth it.

When you are doing the calculations today, remember, we are interested in the *amount of change* in your activity level between weeks, not in the absolute amount of exercises you are able to write down or the absolute number of calories calculated down to the last decimal point. This is not a race against anyone. If you try too hard and pull a muscle, it could backfire—take it easy at first, a small step at a time, and work into a good, regular program.

Do You Understand?

• If you do not understand the value of increased activity, the concept of increased energy expenditure with exercise, or your need for more activity, re-read pages 185–188.

The graph of calories expended in walking and other exercise will serve as a feedback device to let you know if you are burning up more calories this week than last week. Figure out your activity and energy expenditure for last week, fill in the "Calories" on your Daily Activity Sheet, and plot the number of miles per day you walked last week on your Daily Energy Out (activity) Graph. This will be your baseline. Next week you will add to it to see how well you have been able to increase the energy-out (activity) side of the equation.

HOMEWORK.

A. Lesson Eight Food Diary.

B. Lesson Eight Daily Behavior Checklist.

C. Daily Activity Sheet.

D. Daily Energy-Out (activity) Graph.

For Lesson Nine you will need a calorie counter or book that lists the caloric value of various foods. You may find a listing in one of your cookbooks. They can also be purchased at any bookstore and in many markets and drug stores, or by sending one dollar to the Superintendent of Documents, U.S. Government Printing Office, Washington, D.C. 20402, and asking for Agriculture Information Bulletin No. 364, "Calories and Weight."

FOOD DIARY – Lesson Eight

Day of Week _____   Name_____

Time	M/S	H	Location of Eating	Food Type and Quantity
6:00				
11:00				
4:00				
9:00				

FOOD DIARY – Lesson Eight

Day of Week _____   Name_____

Time	M/S	H	Location of Eating	Food Type and Quantity
6:00				
11:00				
4:00				
9:00				

FOOD DIARY – Lesson Eight

Day of Week _____   Name_____

Time	M/S	H	Location of Eating	Food Type and Quantity
6:00				
11:00				
4:00				
9:00				

FOOD DIARY – Lesson Eight

Day of Week _____   Name_____

Time	M/S	H	Location of Eating	Food Type and Quantity
6:00				
11:00				
4:00				
9:00				

FOOD DIARY – Lesson Eight

Day of Week _____   Name_____

Time	M/S	H	Location of Eating	Food Type and Quantity
6:00				
11:00				
4:00				
9:00				

FOOD DIARY – Lesson Eight

Day of Week _____   Name_____

Time	M/S	H	Location of Eating	Food Type and Quantity
6:00				
11:00				
4:00				
9:00				

FOOD DIARY – Lesson Eight

Day of Week _____   Name_____

Time	M/S	H	Location of Eating	Food Type and Quantity
6:00				
11:00				
4:00				
9:00				

DAILY BEHAVIOR CHECKLIST — Lesson 8

Points: Most of the time, or yes = 3
          Sometimes   = 2
          Not at all, or no   = 1

	Days of the Week						
	1	2	3	4	5	6	7
1. *Daily Checklist* a. Morning review							
b. Evening scoring							
2. *Food Diary* a. Recording my food							
3. *Cue Elimination – I* a. Designated eating place							
b. Food stored in opaque container							
4. *Pre-planning* a. Pre-plan one or more meals or snacks							
b. Shop from a prepared list							
5. *Cue Elimination – II* a. Leave food behind on the plate							
b. Split large meals into seconds							
c. Throw away or label leftovers							
d. Don't accept food from others							
6. *Energy Use* a. Record miles walked per day							
b. Increase miles walked per day							
c. Increase other activities							
DAILY TOTALS							

Total Points for the Week _____   Weight _____

DAILY ACTIVITY SHEET

(Fill in miles per day walked and minutes of exercise or extra activities)

	Monday		Tuesday		Wednesday		Thursday		Friday		Saturday		Sunday	
	Miles	Calories	Miles	Calories	Miles	Calories	Miles	Calories	Miles	Calories	Miles	Calories	Miles	Calories
Miles Walked														
	Mins.	Calories	Mins.	Calories	Mins.	Calories	Mins.	Calories	Mins.	Calories	Mins.	Calories	Mins.	Calories
Activity or Exercise														

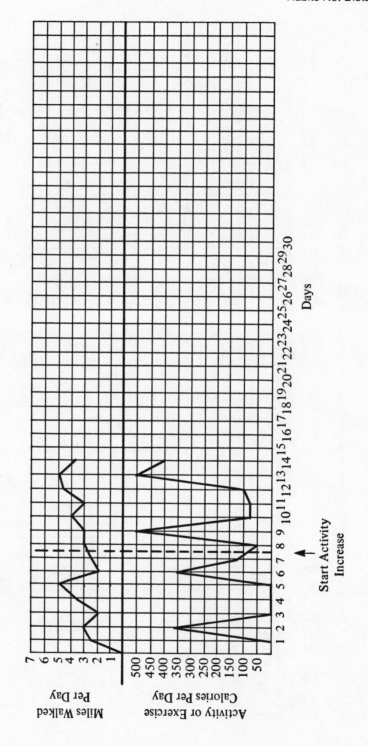

DAILY ENERGY-OUT (ACTIVITY) GRAPH

SAMPLE

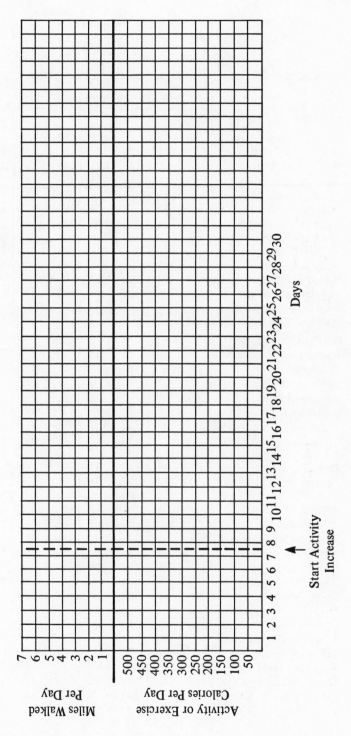

DAILY ENERGY-OUT (ACTIVITY) GRAPH

CALORIES BURNED UP DURING TEN MINUTES OF CONTINUOUS ACTIVITY

	Body Wt.#	150#	175#	200#	225#	250#	275#	300#
LOCOMOTION								
Walking - 2 mph		35	40	46	53	58	64	69
One mile - @ 2 mph		105	120	140	157	175	193	210
Walking - 4-1/2 mph		67	78	87	98	110	120	131
One mile - @ 4-1/2 mph		89	103	115	130	147	160	173
Walking Upstairs		175	201	229	259	288	318	350
Walking Downstairs		67	78	88	100	111	122	134
Jogging - 5-1/2 mph		108	127	142	160	178	197	215
Running - 7 mph		141	164	187	208	232	256	280
Running - 12 mph (sprint)		197	230	258	295	326	360	395
Running in place (140 count)		242	284	325	363	405	447	490
Bicycle - 5-1/2 mph		50	58	67	75	83	92	101
Bicycle - 13 mph		107	125	142	160	178	197	216
RECREATION								
Badminton or Vollyball		52	67	75	85	94	104	115
Baseball (except pitcher)		47	54	62	70	78	86	94
Basketball		70	82	93	105	117	128	140
Bowling (nonstop)		67	82	90	100	111	122	133
Canadian Airforce								
Exercise -0.5 Bx 1A		83	97	108	123	137	152	168
2A		104	122	137	155	173	190	207
3A,4A		147	170	192	217	244	267	290
5A,6A		167	192	217	240	270	300	330
Dancing - moderate		42	49	55	62	69	77	86
Dancing - vigorous		57	67	75	86	94	104	115
Square Dancing		68	80	90	103	113	124	135
Football		83	97	110	123	137	152	167
Golf - foursome		40	47	55	62	68	75	83
Horseback Riding (trot)		67	78	90	102	112	123	134
Ping Pong		38	43	52	58	64	71	78
Skiing - (alpine)		96	113	128	145	160	177	195
Skiing - (cross country)		117	137	158	174	194	214	235
Skiing - (water)		73	92	104	117	130	142	165
Swimming - (backstroke)								
20 yd/min		38	43	52	58	64	71	79
Swimming - (breaststroke)								
20 yd/min		48	55	63	72	80	88	96
Swimming - crawl 20 yd/min		48	55	63	72	80	88	96
Tennis		67	80	92	103	115	125	135
Wrestling, Judo or Karate		129	150	175	192	213	235	257

CALORIES BURNED UP DURING TEN MINUTES OF
CONTINUOUS ACTIVITY (Continued)

	Body Wt.#	150#	175#	200#	225#	250#	275#	300#
PERSONAL ACTIVITIES								
Sleeping		12	14	16	18	20	22	24
Sitting (TV or reading)		12	14	16	18	20	22	24
Sitting (Conversing)		18	21	24	28	30	34	37
Washing/Dressing		32	38	42	47	53	58	63
Standing quietly		14	17	19	21	24	26	28
SEDENTARY OCCUPATION								
Sitting/Writing		18	21	24	28	30	34	37
Light Office Work		30	35	39	45	50	55	60
Standing (Light activity)		24	28	32	37	40	45	50
HOUSEWORK								
General Housework		41	48	53	60	68	74	81
Washing Windows		42	49	54	61	69	76	83
Making Beds		39	46	52	58	65	75	85
Mopping Floors		46	54	60	68	75	83	91
Light Gardening		36	42	47	53	59	66	73
Weeding Garden		59	69	78	88	98	109	120
Mowing Grass (power)		41	48	53	60	67	74	81
Mowing Grass (manual)		45	53	58	66	74	81	88
Shoveling Snow		78	92	100	117	130	144	160
LIGHT WORK								
Factory Assembly		24	28	32	37	40	45	50
Truck-Auto Repair		42	49	54	61	69	76	83
Carpentry/Farm Work		38	45	51	58	64	71	78
Brick Laying		34	40	45	51	57	62	67
HEAVY WORK								
Chopping Wood		73	86	96	109	121	134	156
Pick & Shovel Work		67	79	88	100	110	120	130

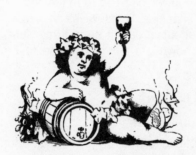

Lesson Nine

Snacks, Cues and Holidays

WEIGH-IN AND HOMEWORK.

Weigh yourself, record your weight, graph your weight change, and check off your Homework.

—Is your Lesson Eight Food Diary complete? Yes_____ No_____

—Did you include pre-planning on the Food Diary? Yes_____ No_____

—Is your Lesson Eight Daily Behavior Checklist filled in? Yes_____ No_____

—Did you record your miles per day on your Daily Activity Sheet? Yes_____ No_____

—Did you graph your miles per day? Yes_____ No_____

207

—Are your minutes per day of activity recorded on your Daily Activity Sheet? Yes—————— No——————

For today's lesson, you need a calorie counter.

REVIEW: PRE-PLANNING.

After the five-week Maintenance period you began to work with pre-planning, one of the most difficult but most effective tools in the program. The concept of pre-planning cannot be emphasized or repeated enough. If you can determine what you are going to eat one or two meals in the future, *by habit,* you will be freed from the decision-making that results in impulse eating or snacking. Housewives are usually best at pre-planning and find it a most effective eating control measure. Several psychology experiments have shown pre-planning alone to be an effective weight control technique.

How Has It Worked for You?

- Are you still pre-planning? Yes—————— No——————

- Have you noticed any change in your appetite response when something unplanned is offered to you or included in a pre-planned meal? Yes—————— No——————

- Have you pre-planned long enough to sense a difference in impulse eating? Yes—————— No——————

Pre-planning is a technique that becomes easier with time. You will gain increasing control of food encounters as you practice pre-planning.

Cue Elimination

The first set of cue elimination exercises was designed to decrease the strength of the external stimuli that are cues to eat. Everyone is influenced by external cues; when you become aware of them, you can free yourself from them. Because it usually takes several months for a strong cue to fade and become neutral, cue elimination must be practiced constantly. By now you should be able to sense a difference in the strength of external cues for eating.

The second set of cue elimination tasks was as important as the first set: 1. Don't finish everything on your plate! (This command is the only way to free you from a habit most of us were taught as children. Although it may have been defensible at that time, it has persisted in most of us to a time and situation when it is no longer reasonable.) 2.

Don't accept food from others. 3. Try to minimize your contacts with food. 4. Use smaller plates. 5. Throw away or plan a use for leftovers.

All of these cue elimination tasks are designed to set you free, to liberate you from eating habits learned in childhood, Like the cue elimination exercises in the first set, these too must be practiced daily or they will never become habitual.

Some people find it necessary to set aside the food they are going to leave behind at the beginning of a meal, and may go so far as to put it on a separate plate with plastic wrap over it, to make sure it doesn't get eaten. Leaving food behind is a hard habit to develop. But it will pay off whenever you are confronted with large portions that are beyond your caloric needs. This occurs regularly at restaurants, in social situations, and at home when you find you are eating but not really hungry.

Energy: Its Use and Abuse

During the last two lessons you have learned about activity and how to use more energy than you consume. Even though exercise does not seem worth it at times (the loneliest sport in the world, jogging, only burns up ten Calories per minute), it has a cumulative value: One extra mile walked each day is worth almost a pound a month, or 12 pounds in a year. A greater rate of energy expenditure will accelerate your weight loss, and it may reestablish a losing trend if you have reached a plateau. Your muscle and cardiovascular tone will improve, your weight loss will be primarily from stored fat, and your hunger will be blunted or even eliminated by vigorous exercise. Finally, exercise often helps people overcome cues for over-eating, like boredom and the blues. Exercise and increased activity work *together* to shift the energy equation out of balance. You start using that energy stored as fat.

Last week you kept track of your walking mileage and also your activities each day. The goal was a 50 percent increase in the distance walked, and an increase of at least 50 Calories per day in other activities.

How Did You Do?

- Did you keep track of your mileage? Yes_____ No_____
- Were you able to increase your mileage by 50 percent? Yes_____ No_____
- What tricks did you use to accomplish this?

    1. _____

    2. _____

    3. _____

(Example: "I used the most distant phone." "I parked at the far end of the parking lot.")

- Were you able to add some form of exercise to your daily routine? Yes_____ No_____

- What kinds of exercises were you able to introduce?

    1. _____

    2. _____

    3. _____

For next week keep walking at this week's level, or increase it, and try to increase your daily energy expenditure through exercise by at least 50 Calories. Remember, exercise is much easier to do with someone else. If you have a social commitment to exercise with someone, the chances are much greater that you will do the exercise than if your commitment is only in private to yourself.

NEW TOPIC: SNACKS AND HOLIDAY CONTROL (EATING WITH INFORMED CONSENT).

Snacks are usually eaten in response to psychological, not physiological hunger. The hunger pangs that lead to snacking are almost always triggered by environmental stimuli. These hunger cues are situation specific and time limited. In other words, if you move away from the situation, or don't respond to the cues by eating, the feeling of hunger will go away.

For example, imagine yourself walking down the street on a sunny morning, thinking about the coming weekend with a day off from work. Suddenly, you pass a bakery shop. The sight of fresh pastries in the window and the smell from the open door are very powerful cues. They cause you to react with a sensation of hunger—even though ten seconds before you had no thoughts of food or hunger. If you remove yourself rapidly from the situation, the hunger will fade away. Or, if you don't leave, but stand in front of the shop in the presence of the cues long enough without responding to them (by eating), the hunger will also go away.

Snacking may not be a problem for you at this point. However, there are two situations where it may reemerge. The first is during vacations or holidays, where the environment is saturated with food. The second is the snacking that occurs in the context of an ordinary meal. There is no difference between eating that larger dessert or third piece of chicken now, "because it is on the table," and having it as a snack later, "because it is in the refrigerator."

Only eat what you need—leave the rest on the table. If you can control the impulse to eat when you are not hungry, you will dramatically decrease your caloric intake without depriving yourself or feeling hungry.

As we have discussed, hunger pangs usually are induced by stimuli in your environment. One type of example was given above, where you feel a pang of hunger when you suddenly see some attractive food, even though you were not thinking about eating. Another type of cue is found in the chains of associations that lead to eating. To give one example of an association chain: On a Sunday drive, you see a perfectly shaped pine tree which reminds you of Christmas, which recalls the memory of childhood Christmases and the turkey dinner that mother used to make, which in turn, makes you feel hungry. If you weren't aware of this progression of associations, you might pull over at the next Howard Johnson's—but by recognizing the cause of your hunger, you would be able to combat it more effectively.

You have learned a great number of snack inhibiting techniques in the past eight lessons, some of which will be appropriate to almost any situation. Although they were introduced in different contexts, they will be your first line of defense during holidays and vacations. With some reflection you can see how to apply them to impulse eating in any situation. The techniques most commonly used to combat impulses are:

1. Introduce an eating delay. Set a timer when you feel hungry and have your snack only after you have waited a pre-determined amount of time. Progressively increase the length of time before your snack.

2. If you snack, put the food down between bites, take longer to eat the snack, and enjoy the food. If you permit yourself to do this, you won't feel guilty about eating, and you will tend to eat less over a longer period of time.

3. Snack only at your Designated Appropriate Eating Place.

4. Substitute alternate activities for eating. Either modify the behavior chain that leads to eating, while the impulse is still remote from food, or, when you are actually confronted with the snack, substitute an incompatible behavior or a low-calorie snack food.

5. Pre-plan your food intake to decrease the strength of your impulses.

6. Only buy foods on a full stomach, and avoid buying snack foods for future use.

7. Leave some behind—part of a cookie, a piece of popcorn, a bite of cake. When you are finished, throw it away.

In other words, control your environment. Don't let it control you!

**How Do You Feel About Your
Progress with These Techniques?**

- Do you remember the cue elimination techniques just mentioned?
  Yes_____ No_____

- Are you still using them every day? Yes_____ No_____

- Which ones are most useful for your snacks?

  1. _____

  2. _____

  3. _____

- Do you feel like you are beginning to control your environment?
  Yes_____ No_____

You are about to receive some new techniques for your snack prevention program. However, in order to make sense out of them, you need to know more about the physiology of eating and hunger. Several investigators have made basic observations about the biology of hunger that bear directly on impulse eating.[9] They asked individuals who had gone without food for a standard amount of time to drink an entire meal of chocolate liquid through a straw. The subjects could not see into the food container, and they had no external way of knowing how much liquid they were consuming. In addition, they did not know the calorie content of the drink; it could be (and was) varied as much as tenfold before the subjects could taste the difference. In the experiment the liquid always looked, felt, and tasted the same. They simply drank the chocolate-flavored liquid until they felt full.

The results of the experiments were surprising. One psychologist found that subjects drank the same amount of fluid every day, despite marked changes in caloric content. Volume or bulk appeared to be the factor that told people when they were satisfied.

Another psychologist found that belief is a critical variable in the subjective feeling of being full. If subjects believed a liquid meal was high in calories, they were satisfied with less food than if they believed it was low in calories. Like the other study, the actual caloric content of the food was irrelevant. Their conclusions were: *Humans cannot sense the caloric content of food.* People only begin to "feel" hunger after they had been on a low-calorie liquid for several days.

These experiments appear to contradict many current ideas about hunger, for example, the notion that hunger is satisfied by raising your blood sugar. At the present time no one knows how the brain senses "fullness." Volume and belief are not the entire answer, but they are important.

We can make use of the volume sensors in several ways. When you have an overwhelming urge for a snack, make sure it has volume. Precede each snack with a glass of water, a diet drink, or some food with volume and few calories. If it is a conditioned and not a physiological hunger, this will help you ignore the pangs. Eventually whatever is telling you to be hungry will begin to lose its power over you—it will no longer be rewarded with food.

Do You Understand This?

• Can you define hunger? Yes_____ No_____

• Describe where you feel hunger and what it feels like..

_____

_____

_____

• Did you understand the hunger and volume experiments? Yes_____ No_____

• Do you see how bulk can help decrease your hunger sensations? Yes_____ No_____

The volume experiments also suggest a strategy for controlling meals. Include some bulk, either liquid or solid, like a large salad, before you eat your main course. This will provide the internal sensation of satiety sooner than if you eat in the reverse order.

The technique of incorporating bulk in your diet *must* be used in conjunction with the techniques we introduced previously. There is no reason to inhibit your hunger response unless you are developing the habit of eating only in response to hunger. To put it another way, there is little point in working on your hunger by eating your salad first, if you still feel compelled to eat everything on your plate, or if you still eat everything because your attention is drawn away by another activity like reading.

A second technique for snacking is food substitution: using low-calorie foods for snacks. Sometimes you will crave caviar. When that happens, you should have it and enjoy it. Don't worry about the calories. At other times, you may be satisfied with something low in calories. Part of your decision will be made on the basis of how many calories you think there are in foods available to you. If you are given a choice between duck and lobster at a fancy party, there is no intuitive way to know what the caloric content of either one is. If you are tired of duck, you might choose lobster by chance for variety. However, if you know that there are only 95 Calories in 3½ ounces, you might decide to save 250 Calories by having it instead of the same amount of duck.

Since the caloric content of foods is not intuitively obvious, effective snack substitution depends on caloric knowledge. We have included some snack hints with today's materials, to help you look at the caloric content of impulse foods and to help you at critical points—when you are at a party, buffet, reception, or looking for something to nibble on at home. Knowledge about the relative calories will help you make your decision. This information will be most helpful when there are equally tempting choices. Last week you were to buy a small inexpensive calorie counter. Your task now is to list the snacks you recorded on your Food Diary last week, on the Snack Worksheet in the homework materials for this week. Choose an alternate snack from the calorie book. Figure out your savings by subtracting the calories in the substitute snack from the calories in the original snack.

Are There Still Some Questions?

- Do you still have questions about how to use bulk to combat hunger? Yes_____ No_____
  (Although it may not be effective all of the time, it will be effective enough of the time to help you cut down on your total intake.)

- Do you see how this technique could be used before a party? Yes_____ No_____

- Do you see how some knowledge of snack calories fits into this program? Yes_____ No_____

- Do you understand how to use the Snack Worksheet?

In summary, you have reviewed all of the tools presented to you during the first eight lessons, which can help you deal with snacks. They may not be as relevant at the present time as they will be during a vacation or holiday. Remember, however, that these techniques are easier to practice now. Later you will be confronted with an overwhelming array of foods, hor d'oeuvres, birthday and Christmas goodies, etc., and it will be much harder to remember your new coping skills at the height of temptation.

The Food Diaries will be optional for the next two weeks. Copies will be included among your materials for each week; use the Food Diary if you still find it helpful. At this point, most people begin phasing Food Diaries out of their daily routine, replacing them with a Daily Maintenance Checklist. Some people find the Food Diary so useful that they prefer to use it indefinitely, while others find them unnecessarily time consuming by this point and would rather use the simpler form.

A *Maintenance Behavior Checklist* is included for you to use each day. It should be used two ways. First, use it as a memory aid to remind you of your new behaviors *before* you eat. To properly use it in this way, you should read it before every meal. This will establish a mental framework for you when you start to eat, and you will tend to carry out the relevant behaviors on the checklist because they will be fresh in your mind. The second use of the Checklist is for recording and self-evaluation. Every evening check off the relevant boxes to rate your day's performance. When you see a line of boxes without an entry, ask yourself, "Why?" If you feel you need to improve, go back to the lesson where that particular technique was covered and relearn it. Try to use the Checklist in both ways—as a reminder to use your new eating skills, and as a feedback device to keep track of how well you are doing.

HOMEWORK.

A. Continue to fill in the Daily Activity Sheet for the coming week. Try to reach 250 Calories of energy used up above your baseline every day. This will be the *combined* total energy spent in walking and other forms of exercising.

B. Fill in your Daily Energy-Out Graph (with the Lesson Eight homework forms) with information from your Daily Activity sheet.

C. Fill in the Snack Worksheet.

D. Fill in the Maintenance Behavior Checklist every day.

E. The Food Diary is optional.

FOOD DIARY – Lesson Nine
(OPTIONAL)

Day of Week _____   Name _____

Time	M/S	H	Food Type and Quantity
6:00			
11:00			
4:00			
9:00			

FOOD DIARY – Lesson Nine
(OPTIONAL)

Day of Week _____   Name _____

Time	M/S	H	Food Type and Quantity
6:00			
11:00			
4:00			
9:00			

FOOD DIARY – Lesson Nine
(OPTIONAL)

Day of Week _____   Name _____

Time	M/S	H	Food Type and Quantity
6:00			
11:00			
4:00			
9:00			

FOOD DIARY – Lesson Nine
   (OPTIONAL)

Day of Week _____   Name _____

Time	M/S	H	Food Type and Quantity
6:00			
11:00			
4:00			
9:00			

FOOD DIARY – Lesson Nine
(OPTIONAL)

Day of Week _____   Name _____

Time	M/S	H	Food Type and Quantity
6:00			
11:00			
4:00			
9:00			

FOOD DIARY – Lesson Nine
(OPTIONAL)

Day of Week _____   Name _____

Time	M/S	H	Food Type and Quantity
6:00			
11:00			
4:00			
9:00			

FOOD DIARY – Lesson Nine
    (OPTIONAL)

Day of Week _____   Name _____

Time	M/S	H	Food Type and Quantity
6:00			
11:00			
4:00			
9:00			

SNACK WORKSHEET

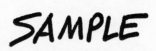

For This Food	Substitute	Savings
EXAMPLE. CAVIAR, 3.5 OZ. - 316 CAL.	CRAB MEAT, 3.5 OZ 93 CAL.	223 CAL.
DUCK, 3.5 OZ. - 350 CAL.	LOBSTER MEAT, 3.5 OZ 95 CAL.	255 CAL.
BEER-(SCHLITZ, 12 OZ) 150 CAL	BEER (MILLER LITE) 12 OZ 90 CAL	54 CAL.
HOSTESS TWINKIE 144 CAL	2-SUNSHINE FIG BARS 90 CAL	54 CAL.

SNACK WORKSHEET

For This Food	Substitute	Savings

SNACK HINTS

1. Make snacks hard to get. They should require preparation, like popcorn, or be hard to eat, like frozen bananas.

2. Try to avoid extremes of intake—neither starvation nor overeating. They both lead to feast/ famine cycles, and extra eating between meals. Never skip a meal if you're hungry—eat with control.

3. High protein foods will decrease food cravings—they last longer.

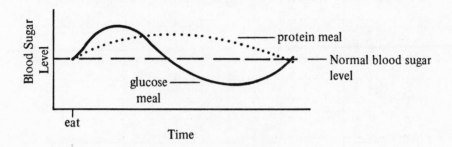

4. A small glass of unsweetened fruit juice will help you overcome that famished feeling— combine it with a high protein snack if necessary.

5. Tea and coffee (even decaffinated) stimulate stomach secretions and hunger.

6. Alcohol is caloric, stimulates hunger, and leads to higher levels of blood triglycerides.

7. Read labels. Some artificial creamers use coconut (saturated fat) oils instead of corn oil and may contain more calories. Diet colas vary from nearly zero to 35 calories per can. Water-packed foods have many fewer calories than syrup-packed. The order in which contents are listed on labels indicate how much of each is present inside the container. For example—the Cheerios label says it contains oat flower, wheat starch, sugar, salt, sodium phosphate. Sugar is the third most prevalent constituent of Cheerios.

8. Carry a low-calorie sweetner with you.

9. If quantity is your weakness, add bulk; for example, raw vegetables, long grain rice, a diet soda before dinner, or starting dinner with boullion for a soup course.

10. Keep in mind that one mixed drink like a margarita is roughly calorically equal to a Hershey Bar, or a creme-filled cupcake.

11. Try to always have an alternate response to snack eating—and keep in mind, a little hunger is the feeling of losing weight.

DAILY ACTIVITY SHEET

(Fill in miles per day walked and minutes of exercise or extra activities)

	Monday		Tuesday		Wednesday		Thursday		Friday		Saturday		Sunday	
	Miles	Calories	Miles	Calories	Miles	Calories	Miles	Calories	Miles	Calories	Miles	Calories	Miles	Calories
Miles Walked														
	Mins.	Calories	Mins.	Calories	Mins.	Calories	Mins.	Calories	Mins.	Calories	Mins.	Calories	Mins.	Calories
Activity or Exercise														

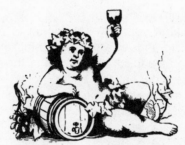

Lesson Ten

Environmental Support— Family and Friends

WEIGH-IN AND HOMEWORK.

Weigh yourself, record your weight and graph your weight change.

My total weight loss for the past fourteen weeks is _____ .

Homework.

—I completed my Daily Activity Sheet? Yes_____
No_____

—I filled in my Maintenance Behavior Checklist every day?
Yes_____ No_____

—I completed my Optional Food Diary? Yes_____
No_____

227

SOCIAL ENVIRONMENT.

The first nine learning weeks of this program have been devoted to techniques that have been largely individual-oriented. The final section of this program describes ways of interacting with your immediate social environment. The people around you have an important role in helping you control your weight and maintain your new eating behavior patterns. The first step in interacting with the people around you in a new way—in a way that helps you lose weight—will be to tell them about the material that will be presented in this chapter: read it to them, describe it to them, or let them read it for themselves. These ideas are for your entire household . . . for everyone around you. If you only work on changing your behaviors, without involving those around you in your program, it won't be nearly as effective.

Your social environment, your spouse, family, and friends, are the people most influential in your life. This group of people provides your source of reinforcement and rewards: they compliment you, notice your changes, and give you feedback in the form of their opinions. The more they know about this program, the better. Some of the new behaviors we have taught you may have seemed odd or even silly at first, like not watching television while eating, putting your fork down between bites, and changing places at the table. When people in your social environment know the reasons for these changes and support you, they will seem less silly, and the program will be more effective.

One of the strategies we introduced in the first lesson was to have you teach the content of each weekly lesson to someone else. The advantage of this technique is that when you think it through, review the various procedures, and teach someone else, it helps you learn the material. If you have made a regular practice of teaching someone else, you are way ahead.

Many times in this text the point has been made that *no one is to blame* for obesity. Eating is a learned behavior like all other behaviors, and there should be neither moral value nor stigma attached to it. There is no blame to fix. The point now is to maximize the chance of your successfully maintaining your new behaviors, and the best way is by involving others.

REVIEW: ACTIVITY.

Three weeks ago you learned about the basic energy equation:

ENERGY IN (food) = ENERGY USED (activity) + STORAGE (fat)

or,

$$FAT = FOOD - ACTIVITY$$

This relationship between energy and matter is true for the whole universe: there are no exceptions. Working on increasing the energy-used part of the equation has many advantages. Last week your goal was an increase of 250 Calories per day above your baseline caloric expenditure. This is equivalent to 1750 Calories, or one-half pound extra weight loss for the week. You were to accomplish this increase by walking more every day, as measured by a pedometer, and by incorporating some extra activity into your daily routine.

Have You Done What You Set Out to Do?

- Did you understand the assignment? Yes_____ No_____ (Page 168)

- Did you achieve the goal? Yes_____ No_____

- Are you walking at least 50 percent above your baseline? Yes_____ No_____

- What ways are you using to increase your walking?

  1. _____

  2. _____

  3. _____

- What activities have you added to your weekly routine?

  1. _____

  2. _____

  3. _____

REVIEW: SNACKS, CUES, AND HOLIDAYS (EATING WITH INFORMED CONSENT).

Last week you reviewed many of the techniques introduced during the first eight weeks to control impulse eating or snacking. These techniques are successful because hunger pangs are usually a reflex response to external cues which are not related to a physiological need for food. These impulses to eat are time limited; if you do not respond to them, they will go away. Every time you are able to "wait out" an impulse to eat, the cue will become weaker. Each time that particular cue occurs and is not rewarded with food, its strength will decrease and it will provoke a reduced hunger response, until it eventually becomes neutral. You are probably aware at this point of several environmental cues, like television, that have become neutral—they no longer provoke hunger.

Although snacks are under control for most people at this point in the program, there is a tendency for snacking to reemerge during holidays and vacations, when the environment is saturated with food cues and large meals, and when pleasure is the order of the day. These meals often include a snack added to a regular meal. You can recognize it by the rationalizations that allow you to eat a little bit more than you really need; for example, an extra piece of chicken "because it is there on the table," or a large piece of cake because "someone has to eat it." Many times you can counteract the urge to snack by simply asking yourself the question, "Am I hungry?" If the answer is "no," then you should try to pass up the food.

The two new concepts introduced last week were: first, the use of bulk, e.g., a salad or a glass of water, to provide the sensation of satiety earlier in a meal or snack, and second, the use of caloric information. You need to know the calorie content of foods so you can make an informed decision about what to eat. You bought a calorie counter and used it with the Snack Worksheet to give yourself some information about impulse foods. The caloric content of foods is not intuitively obvious, and this is especially true of snack foods, which usually are presented in a situation where you have choices. If you know the caloric content of the foods you are offered, it is easy to choose the one with fewer calories. For now the only calories you should be counting are those needed to do the exercises, and those in snacks. The latter are important because we want you to be able to make conscious informed choices between foods.

How Have You Been Doing?

- Did you look up the caloric value of your snack foods? Yes_____ No_____

- Were you able to substitute snack foods and save calories? Yes_____ No_____

- Were you able to use bulk to decrease your hunger? Yes_____ No_____

- What kinds of bulk?

1. _____

2. _____

3. _____

GENERAL REVIEW—FOR YOU AND THOSE
AROUND YOU (YOUR SOCIAL ENVIRONMENT).

There are many ways to lose weight: diets, drugs, hypnosis, psychotherapy, surgery, medication, shots, etc. All of these are effective for some people, or at least for a while. However, even when they work initially, they are time limited, and usually fail in the long run.

What does *not* happen with these weight control techniques is learning. At the end of the diet or pills you resume eating the way you did before you lost weight, and you usually regain the weight you lost— nothing is accomplished.

The basic assumption in this program is that individuals who are overweight have *learned* to eat in a way that results in too much caloric intake. The basic changes you have made are in behaviors. If you change the circumstances and act of eating (your eating behaviors), you will lose weight.

Eating behavior change is a slow, tedious procedure, and the weight loss results may not be very dramatic. But there are real advantages to this type of program: It does not matter how you came to be overweight; if you can control your eating behaviors, you will be able to lose weight. If you are able to develop new eating habits, your old habits will simply fade away. This is most obvious where the new habit competes with the old ones. For example, eating slowly is incompatible with finishing dinner in three minutes. The only way to make significant eating behavior change is to attack the behaviors systematically, one at a time, and to make changes *even though that particular behavior may not seem relevant to your problem.*

Changing any habit is hard, especially one as old as eating. Change takes time and careful planning, and it has to be approached a step at a time. Very small steps can give a high probability of success. Weight loss is a long-term project and has to be approached on that basis. The rewards of weight loss are distant: looking nice, feeling better, having people compliment you, etc. The rewards of eating are immediate—the taste and texture of food, the visual stimulation, and the feeling of contentment. The difference makes these behaviors difficult to control, but not impossible.

Lesson One concerned the Food Diary, a way of recording behavioral data and quantifying it. The Food Diary is a behavior change technique designed to make you more aware of everything you eat and of the behaviors that accompany your eating: where you eat, whom you eat with, what you do when you're eating, whether or not you are hungry, what you are feeling, and the actual content of the meals. Many times being aware of meal content and the conditions surrounding a meal will give some clues about why you over-eat; for example, eating when you are not hungry, eating when you are watching a particular program on television, or when you are angry, or bored, or sleepy.

Research has shown that overweight people are more sensitive to cues in their environment than thin individuals. These cues may be direct, like the sight of food, or they may be things only secondarily connected with food, things like (1) *objects,* e.g., the refrigerator; (2) *places,* e.g., the kitchen; (3) *situations,* e.g., watching T-V; and (4) *times,* e.g., 3:00 in the afternoon. All of these have been associated in your past with eating, but *not* necessarily with hunger. These stimuli have gained the ability to elicit the feeling that you should eat, whether or not you are hungry, through long-paired association with food.

You practiced a series of exercises designed to eliminate many of the external cues that have been telling you to eat. These included eating in one place, eliminating food from non-food places in the house, putting food in opaque containers, and keeping serving dishes off the table. You also began shopping from a specific list after a full meal, and only eating when eating.

A second set of cue elimination techniques was introduced to decrease the power of cues intrinsic to the food itself. This included not finishing meals, dividing large meals into multiple portions, using smaller plates, throwing away leftovers or committing them to a specific use, and not accepting food from others.

In another lesson you introduced delays into the process of eating. The purpose of this technique was to make meals last longer and give you enough time to enjoy what you eat. If you eat slowly and allow yourself to experience the pleasurable sensations of food without feeling guilty, paradoxically you will eat less. Guilt makes you eat faster and not pay attention to what you are eating. Your food is just consumed; it vanishes and is not experienced.

You spent a whole lesson on techniques for spotting eating problems with the Food Diary and the Behavioral Analysis Form, and taught yourself how to design behavioral solutions for eating behavior problems. These individual problems have varied, from eating too many potato chips while drinking beer (squash the bag of chips to make them less desirable!), to eating cake and cookies when the children come home from school (fix them low-calorie snacks ahead of time—children can be talked into any kind of snacking).

After a five-week Maintenance period you began pre-planning, a key technique that is often difficult without family support. When you can predict your food intake and stick to your predictions, you can avoid impulse eating. Your predictions have to be fairly accurate or you get discouraged—it does not help to continually predict steak and wind up with hot dogs.

The last two topics in the program have already been discussed: systematically increasing activity to burn up more calories, and using a variety of techniques to resist the snacking.

Is Your Family Involved Supportively?

- If you have any questions about any part of the program, turn back to the lesson in which it was presented and review it in greater detail.

- Have your family members tried the behavior change techniques you have been learning? Yes_____ No_____

- Do you think they appreciate the amount of work and effort that goes into modifying a behavior as basic as eating? Yes_____ No_____

- Has anyone in your family or among your friends lost weight as a result of your effort? Yes_____ No_____

NEW TOPIC: THE SOCIAL ENVIRONMENT— SPOUSE, FAMILY, AND FRIENDS.

Families, spouses, and groups of friends have different styles of reacting to someone losing weight. However, there seem to be some patterns of interaction that are common. Interactions that are painful to the person who is trying to lose can be avoided, if they are anticipated and strategies are worked out in advance for coping with them. These interactions do not occur because people are bad, evil, or mean. They occur because the people involved are not fully conscious of them or the harmful effect they can have. They are an habitual way of interacting, and they persist because there has never been sufficient reason to learn a new way to interact.

Some of the most common feelings, through the eyes of the person trying to lose weight, are:

1. "No one seems to be interested in what I'm doing or in changing their own habits; others have bad eating habits and do not seem to care."

2. "My attempts to change are not supported; they are even ridiculed. Often people say the wrong things. They do not mean to hurt my feelings, but they do."

3. "I am discouraged, belittled, made to feel different, and even the brunt of jokes. People tease me about my weight even though I am changing and losing; it makes me want to say 'what the hell' . . ."

4. "My efforts to change are ignored; my family and friends are always pessimistic, often despite my success."

5. "My loss of weight is praised, but when I try to maintain my weight loss and behavior change, they seem to forget and withdraw their support."

6. "I feel like I am being sabotaged; it is obvious to me, but I can't do anything about it:

    a. They give me high-calorie treats and presents;

    b. They insist I have high-calorie treats for them or the children;

    c. They continue the pattern: Togetherness is an evening out with a good meal; we cannot be together without food;

    d. They bring me food at inappropriate times, e.g., while I am watching T-V;

    e. They use food as a sign of affection; it puts me in a bind;

    f. They say I'm becoming too skinny or unhealthy."

The reasons for these reactions are numerous. We can only guess about them. Some family members may not want to have to match your self-control, especially if they weigh too much themselves. They may not want things to change. They may be afraid that when you look nicer you will go away, or they won't have anything to complain about. However, the most probable explanation is that this is the only way they have learned to interact with you when you are losing weight. It is a way that has worked in the past. It is a type of behavior neither one of you has been fully aware of. Fortunately, it is a behavior that is quite amenable to change.

To break out of these stereotyped interactions, the person losing weight—**you**—must take control of the situation. The people around you cannot really read your mind; they have to be told what you want. After all you are altering the relationship by losing weight, looking different, and feeling different about yourself. They need to know how to give you feedback and praise. So—

Ask for support.

Ask for praise. A compliment at the right time will go further than any material reward, be it money or cream puffs.

Ask for feedback and thank them for it.

Remember, many of the behaviors you are changing are hard to detect. Many of your new habits are "non-behaviors," like not eating fast or not eating in many different places. People around you will not intuitively know to compliment you for eating less or not finishing everything on your plate, unless they know your goals. If this program is to succeed, and if you expect to lose weight and maintain that weight loss, then those behaviors must have positive consequences. They have to pay off! You must feel like it has been worth it. If your family and friends have been directly involved in the process of your weight loss, your success is also their success. Your mutual life will be better, and probably longer.

The following suggestions are designed to help you involve others in the Maintenance part of your behavior change program, to make sure that weight loss and Maintenance pay off for you:

1. Ask for what you want—praise, feedback, cooperation, and rewards.

2. Request help with the techniques—those close to you can remind you of them or even experiment with them. Be in it together. If you practice together, you will do better.

3. Request that affection and sharing *not* be in terms of food. You may appreciate a huge gooey chocolate cake for your birthday, but other gifts are more appropriate. When you are offered a "food gift," you are put in a difficult situation. How can you turn down the gift without feeling like you are turning down the affection also? Try to establish the habit of using non-food treats, like flowers or activities, for celebrations.

4. Request that no one in your environment offer you food at any time. They should assume that if you want food, you will ask for it. Being offered food is a very strong social cue for eating—we all feel bad saying "no."

5. Try to minimize food topics in your conversation with friends and family during your period of weight loss. Discuss the program and progress, but request that they not talk about food. Talk about the office picnic or a good recipe are cues for eating.

6. Try to entertain without high-calorie foods. This takes cooperation from everyone. Friends will still visit you despite the lack of potato chips. If they want food, have low-calorie snacks available.

7. If your husband, children, or other significant person eats or snacks a great deal of the time, ask them to try not to do it around you. Watching someone else eat is a very strong cue to eat.

8. Try to develop exercise programs with another person. Companionship makes exercise more fun, makes it a social commitment to exercise, and gives you a non-food social activity.

Do You See the Importance of These Points?

- Do you see the importance of support by family and friends for your behavior change program? Yes_____ No_____
- Do you understand that no one is to blame for these patterns of interaction, that these are just habits which have developed over the years? Yes_____ No_____
- Did any of the common interpersonal reactions sound familiar? Yes_____ No_____
- Do you run into additional patterns repeatedly? Yes_____ No_____
- Are there any additional rules that should be added to the list for your social environment? Yes_____ No_____

SUMMARY.

You have something to be proud of. You have worked hard for the past 15 weeks and made it to the end of this program. Now it is up to you to keep working on eating control.

Maintenance is much easier if you have strong environmental support from your family and friends. In this lesson you learned some of the ground rules for establishing that support. If you shared today's lesson with the people who make up your social environment, then you have greatly increased your chances of maintaining your behavior changes and weight loss.

If you want to analyze your eating behaviors, either now or in the is useful, continue to use it. The only homework in the text for the last five Maintenance weeks is the Maintenance Behavior Checklist. By now the need for other forms of homework is probably fading. The most effective way of using the Maintenance Behavior Checklist is as a cue card and evaluation or feedback device. Read it before each meal, and record your performance at the end of the day.

If you want to analyze your eating behaviors either now or in the future, keep a detailed Food Diary for one week. Use the same form you used for Lesson One (and make additional copies as you need them). When it is completed, turn back to Lesson Six and fill in the remaining half of the Behavioral Analysis Form. This will give you a good picture of how well your behaviors are being maintained, and what areas need improvement.

PAYBACK—THE CONTINGENT
REFUND TO YOURSELF.

It is time for you to reward yourself for completing the homework in the course. Each assignment had a cash value. Although it has not been a great deal of money for each part, cumulatively it has added up to an amount you may care about. The return of the money you have earned is a good way of showing yourself how well you have done in the program.

Add up the amount of money you have earned; it is listed on the Homework Credit Sheet. Take the amount you did not earn and give it away—to your children, your spouse, or to a charity. Take the rest of the money and put it in your pocket—it is yours! Do with it whatever you want. Don't spend it on something for someone else. Don't put it back in the family kitty. You earned it—you spend it.

DAILY BEHAVIOR CHECKLIST – Lesson Ten

Points: Most of the time, or yes = 3
          Sometimes   = 2
          Not at all, or no   = 1

	Days						
	1	2	3	4	5	6	7
1. *Daily Checklist* a. Morning Review							
b. Evening Scoring							
2. *Food Diary* a. Recording my food							
3. *Cue Elimination – I* a. Designated eating place							
b. Only eating when eating							

4. *Eating Delay*
   a. Swallow each forkful before
      adding the next							

5. *Behavior Chains*
   a. Substitute an activity for
      eating							

6. *Pre-planning*
   a. Pre-plan one or more meals or
      snacks							

b. Shop on a full stomach							

7. *Cue Elimination – II*
   a. Use smaller plates when
      possible							

b. Leave food behind on the plate							
c. Split large meals into seconds							
d. Throw away or commit leftovers							
e. Don't accept food from others							
f. Minimize your contact with food.							
Daily Totals							

Total Points for the Week _____   Weight _____

SAMPLE

MAINTENANCE BEHAVIOR CHECKLIST – WEEK _____

✓ : Good Job

	Wt.	Days						
	198	1	2	3	4	5	6	7
Designated eating place		✓	✓	✓	✓	✓	✓	✓
No other activity while eating		✓	✓	✓	✓	✓	✓	
Utensils down between mouthfuls		✓	✓	✓	✓	✓	✓	✓
Smaller plates and shallow bowls		✓	✓		✓		✓	
Leave food behind		✓	✓	✓		✓	✓	
Dispose of (or pre-plan) leftovers		✓	✓	✓	✓	✓		✓
Store food out of sight		✓	✓	✓	✓	✓	✓	✓
Minimize contact with food			✓	✓	✓	✓	✓	✓
Substitute activities for eating		✓	✓	✓	✓	✓	✓	✓
Increase exercise		✓	✓				✓	✓
Increase walking		✓	✓	✓	✓	✓	✓	✓
Pre-plan meals & snacks		✓		✓	✓	✓	✓	✓
Only eat what you need!		✓	✓	✓	✓	✓	✓	
Take time and enjoy your meals		✓	✓	✓		✓	✓	✓

No. of ✓'s 85

MAINTENANCE BEHAVIOR CHECKLIST — WEEK _____

✓ : Good Job

	Wt.	Days						
		1	2	3	4	5	6	7
Designated eating place								
No other activity while eating								
Utensils down between mouthfuls								
Smaller plates and shallow bowls								
Leave food behind								
Dispose of (or pre-plan) leftovers								
Store food out of sight								
Minimize contact with food								
Substitute activities for eating								
Increase exercise								
Increase walking								
Pre-plan meals & snacks								
Only eat what you need!								
Take time and enjoy your meals								

No. of ✓'s _____

MAINTENANCE BEHAVIOR CHECKLIST — WEEK ___

√ : Good Job

	Wt.	Days						
		1	2	3	4	5	6	7
Designated eating place								
No other activity while eating								
Utensils down between mouthfuls								
Smaller plates and shallow bowls								
Leave food behind								
Dispose of (or pre-plan) leftovers								
Store food out of sight								
Minimize contact with food								
Substitute activities for eating								
Increase exercise								
Increase walking								
Pre-plan meals & snacks								
Only eat what you need!								
Take time and enjoy your meals								

No. of √'s ___

MAINTENANCE BEHAVIOR CHECKLIST – WEEK _____

√ : Good Job

Wt. _____

		Days					
	1	2	3	4	5	6	7
Designated eating place							
No other activity while eating							
Utensils down between mouthfuls							
Smaller plates and shallow bowls							
Leave food behind							
Dispose of (or pre-plan) leftovers							
Store food out of sight							
Minimize contact with food							
Substitute activities for eating							
Increase exercise							
Increase walking							
Pre-plan meals & snacks							
Only eat what you need!							
Take time and enjoy your meals							

No. of √'s _____

MAINTENANCE BEHAVIOR CHECKLIST – WEEK _____

√ : Good Job

	Wt.	Days						
		1	2	3	4	5	6	7
Designated eating place								
No other activity while eating								
Utensils down between mouthfuls								
Smaller plates and shallow bowls								
Leave food behind								
Dispose of (or pre-plan) leftovers								
Store food out of sight								
Minimize contact with food								
Substitute activities for eating								
Increase exercise								
Increase walking								
Pre-plan meals & snacks								
Only eat what you need!								
Take time and enjoy your meals								

No. of √'s _____

MAINTENANCE BEHAVIOR CHECKLIST – WEEK ____

✓ : Good Job

Wt. _____

	Days						
	1	2	3	4	5	6	7
Designated eating place							
No other activity while eating							
Utensils down between mouthfuls							
Smaller plates and shallow bowls							
Leave food behind							
Dispose of (or pre-plan) leftovers							
Store food out of sight							
Minimize contact with food							
Substitute activities for eating							
Increase exercise							
Increase walking							
Pre-plan meals & snacks							
Only eat what you need!							
Take time and enjoy your meals							

No. of ✓'s ____

SAMPLE

MASTER DATA SHEET

Name F. S.
Date 7-18-74
Height 5' 9"

Date	Weight	Weight Change	Total Wt. Change	Av. Gr. Loss
7-18	236¼	—	—	—
7-25	233	-3¼	-3¼	-3
8-1	228½	-4½	-7¾	-5
8-8	228¼	-¼	-8	-7.7
8-15	225¾	-2½	-10½	-10.3
8-22	223	-2¾	-13½	-10.5
8-29	221	-2	-15¼	-13.8
9-5	219	-2	-17¼	-15
9-12	221	+2	-15¼	-15.7
9-19	219	-2	-17¼	-18.8
9-26	219	0	-17¼	-20.3
10-3	214½	-4.5	-21¾	-22.4
10-10	217½	+3	-18¾	-21.4
10-17	214	-3.5	-22¼	-23.3
10-24	213	-1	-23¼	-25.2
10-31	VACATION			27
11-7	219½	+1½	-21¾	-26
11-14	218	+3½	-18¼	-26.5
11-21	214	-4	-22¼	-27
11-28	THANKSGIVING	VACATION		
12-5	213	-1	-23¼	-27

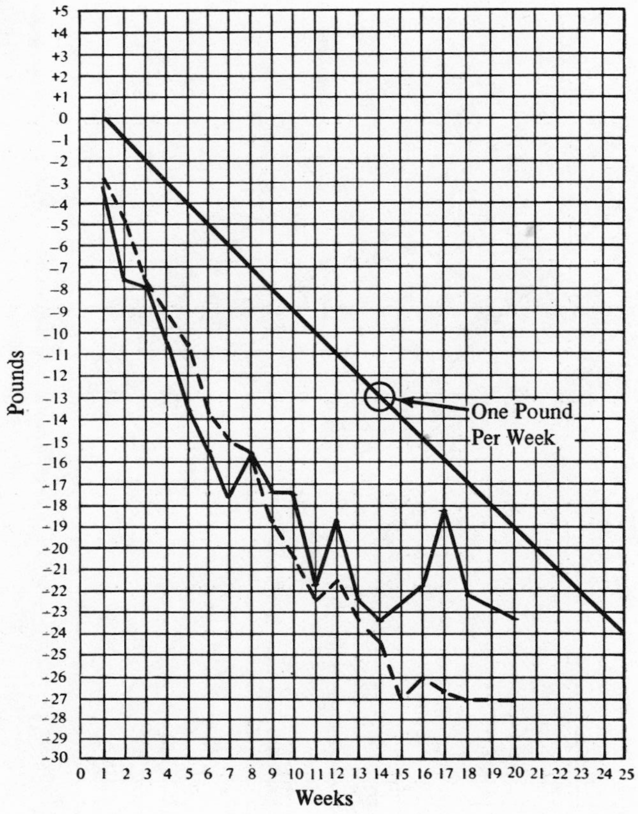

One Pound
Per Week

Pounds

Weeks

0 1 2 3 4 5 6 7 8 9 10 11 12 13 14 15 16 17 18 19 20 21 22 23 24 25

+5 +4 +3 +2 +1 0 -1 -2 -3 -4 -5 -6 -7 -8 -9 -10 -11 -12 -13 -14 -15 -16 -17 -18 -19 -20 -21 -22 -23 -24 -25 -26 -27 -28 -29 -30

MASTER DATA SHEET

Name _____

Date _____

Height _____

Date	Weight	Weight Change	Total Wt Change	Av. Gr. Loss

HOMEWORK CREDIT

Name_____

Lesson	Homework	Refund	Checked by
I.	INTRODUCTION TO THE BEHAVIORAL CONTROL OF WEIGHT.		
	A. Week 1 Food Diary	1.00	
	B. House Plan	1.00	
II.	CUE ELIMINATION		
	A. Week 2 Food Diary	1.50	
	B. Eating Place Record	1.50	
III.	CHANGING THE ACT OF EATING		
	A. Week 3 Food Diary	1.00	
	B. Eating Place Record	.50	
	C. Eating Ratio Column Completed	1.00	
IV.	BEHAVIOR CHAINS AND ALTERNATE ACTIVITIES		
	A. Week 4 Food Diary	.50	
	B. Alternate Activities Specified	.50	
	C. Activity Substitutions Recorded	.50	
	D. One Behavior Chain Defined	.50	
	E. Alternate Link for the Behavior Chain	.50	
V.	PROBLEM SOLVING		
	A. Week 5 Food Diary	.50	
	B. Daily Behavior Checklist	.50	
	C. Eating Place Record	.50	
	D. Eating Ratio Column Completed	.50	
	E. Behavioral Prescription Sheet	.50	
(Maintenance Period):			
M-1	Maintenance Week 1 Food Diary Maintenance Week 1 Behavior Checklist	0.00	
M-2	Maintenance Week 2 Food Diary Maintenance Week 2 Behavior Checklist	0.00	
M-3	Maintenance Week 3 Food Diary Maintenance Week 3 Behavior Checklist	0.00	
M-4	Maintenance Week 4 Food Diary Maintenance Week 4 Behavior Check List	0.00	
M-5	Maintenance Week 5 Food Diary Maintenance Week 5 Behavior Checklist Behavioral Analysis Form (Week 6 and Week 16)	0.00	

HOMEWORK CREDIT

Name _____

Lesson	Homework	Refund	Checked by
VI.	PRE-PLANNING		
	A. Week 6 Food Diary	0.50	
	B. Week 6 Behavior Checklist	1.00	
	C. Pre-planning	1.00	
	D. Behavioral Prescription Sheet	0.50	
VII.	CUE ELIMINATION, PART TWO. ENERGY, PART ONE		
	A. Week 7 Food Diary	0.50	
	B. Week 7 Behavior Checklist	0.50	
	C. Pre-planning	1.00	
	D. Minutes of Exercise by Category and Miles Walked Recorded Daily on the Activity Sheet	1.00	
VIII.	ENERGY USE, PART TWO		
	A. Week 8 Food Diary	0.50	
	B. Maintenance Behavior Checklist	1.00	
	C. Daily Activity Sheet	1.00	
	D. Daily Energy-Out (activity) Graph	1.00	
IX.	SNACKS, CUES AND HOLIDAYS		
	A. Daily Activity Sheet	1.00	
	B. Snack Worksheet	1.00	
	C. Maintenance Behavior Checklist	1.00	
	D. Food Diary (Optional)	–	
X.	ENVIRONMENTAL SUPPORT – FAMILY AND FRIENDS		
	A. Maintenance Behavior Checklist	–	
	B. Food Diary (Optional)	–	
	C. Refund – Total (may be returned at the end of the Final Maintenance Period)	–	

References

1. Stunkard, A.J., New Therapies for the Eating Disorders: Behavior Modification of Obesity and Anorexia Nervosa, *Arch. Gen. Psych., 26:* 391–198, 1972.
2. Schacter, S., and J. Rodin, *Obese Humans and Rats,* Lawrence Erlbaum Associates, Potomac, Maryland, 1974.
3. Schacter, S., and Gross, L.P., Manipulated Time and Eating Behaviors, *Journal of Personality and Social Psychology, 10:* 98–106, 1968.
4. Stewart, S., and Davis, B., *Slim Chance in a Fat World,* Research Press, Champaign, Illinois, 1972, p. 85.
5. Mayer, J., and Bullen, B., Nutrition and Athletic Performance, *Physiological Reviews, 40:* 369–397, 1960.
6. Margen, S., Energy Balance With Increasing Weight, in Wilson, N.L. (ed), *Obesity,* F.A. Davis, Philadelphia, 1969, pp. 77–89.
7. Mayer, J., *Overweight: Causes, Costs, and Control,* Prentice Hall, Englewood Cliffs, New Jersey, 1968, pp. 69–83.
8. Mayer, J., *Overweight: Causes, Costs, and Control, Prentice Hall,* Englewood Cliffs, New Jersey, 1968, p. 79.
9. Wooley, S.C., Physiologic versus Cognitive Factors in Short- Term Food Regulation in the Obese and Nonobese, *Psychosomatic Medicine, 34:* 62–68, 1972.

Bibliography

The individual techniques in this manual have been collected from many sources. In most cases, it is impossible to say who first thought of each individual therapeutic technique, and award credit accordingly. Food diaries, self monitoring, behavioral analysis, increasing activity, decreasing cue saliency, snack substitution, decreasing rate of eating, reinforcement for homework and attendance, feedback about progress, and family interventions are the stock in trade of modern nutritional counseling.

The work of the following investigators in the areas indicated was relied on as source material for this manual.

C.B. Ferster is one of the pioneers in obesity research who looked into the psychological determinants of eating behaviors and proposed the model from which ultimately this program has been derived.

R.L. Hagen has explored the role of bibliotherapy and aversive treatments in weight control programs.

H.A. Jordan has developed materials for use in behavioral weight reduction programs, along with investigating the determinants of hunger and satiety in the thin and obese populations.

L.S. Levitz has worked with weight control program development and self help programs for the obese.

M.J. Mahoney has extensively investigated the cognitive aspects of hunger, eating, and satiety, and has systematically explored the basic postulates underlying the behavioral treatments of obesity.

R.W. Malott and *Behaviordelia, Inc.* provided my introduction to the behavioral techniques of contingency management, behavior chains and alternate activities, and the elements of behavioral analysis.

J.E. Mayer demonstrated much of the basic physiology of eating and the relationship between activity levels and obesity.

W.T. McReynolds has investigated the elements of behavior therapy programs for weight control and has developed stimulus control techniques to the ultimate (e.g., removing light bulbs from patients' refrigerators).

R.E. Nesbett extensively investigated the cognitive aspects of eating behaviors and the cues for hunger and satiety.

S.B. Penick demonstrated the efficacy of behavioral methods and the worth of groups for treating obesity.

L.D. Ross investigated cue saliency and developed some of the common sense "out of sight, out of mind" cue elimination techniques.

S. Schacter devised many brilliant experiments to illustrate the effects of the environment on the eating response in humans.

R.B. Stuart is the experimenter and organizer *par excellence* of the field of obesity and weight control.

A.J. Stunkard has been both an experimenter and key theoretician in weight control for the past twenty-five years.

J.P. Wollersheim was the first person to investigate the effect of a written program like *Learning to Eat* in group therapy situations.

Susan and Orland Wooley have carried out one of the most systematic series of investigations into the mechanisms of hunger, satiety, and eating behavior.

P. Watslowick, J. Haley, S. Minuchin, and *G. Bach* have been my models for family and couple interaction and intervention as described in the final chapter.